"Like an official conducting
novelist Lauren Sanders pluck
and bodies to reveal their hidden lusts, and when all is said and done, nary a body cavity is spared."

–Time Out New York

"This sexy little novel isn't afraid to be steamy–but it isn't too jaded for romance either."

–The Advocate

"Lauren Sanders is a writer of extraordinary skill."

–Bay Area Reporter

"Without wit or heart, this much sex would be unsexy, particularly if the author were using the titillation factor as mere bait for jacket blurbs. Instead, it serves a broader purpose, illustrating that the boundaries we use to demarcate civilized society are largely an illusion, and that labels like 'porn star,' 'cancer patient,' and 'lesbian' are meant to signify–falsely– 'people nothing like us.' Here sex bleeds so naturally into life, and life into sex, that books that shy from this human realm begin to seem prissy and suspect.'

–City Pages (Minneapolis/St. Paul)

"Sanders zips and zooms through Rachel's overturned life with prose as sharp, quick, and deadly as any suicide mission."

–Out Magazine

"The fact that Sanders can so overtly take on sex and death, write almost exclusively of their relationship to each other and their effects on a developing personality, and not sound clichéd, is a monumental achievement in itself."

–Toronto Star

"Kamikaze Lust is a whirl of a New York neurotic fast-quipping with a line or two courtesy of Miss Sandra Bernhardt, but who better to borrow from than the Princess of Pith?"

–Time Out London

lauren sanders

kamikaze lust

Deborah—
A privilege to
read with you.

akashic books
new york

This is a work of fiction. All names, characters, places, and incidents are the product of the author's imagination. Any resemblance to real events or persons, living or dead, is entirely coincidental.

Published by Akashic Books

Cover photo by Howard Levenson
Author photo by Claire Holt
Design and layout by R. Devine

ISBN: 1-888 451-08-4
Library of Congress Catalog Card Number: 99-95534

Third Printing

Akashic Books
PO Box 1456
New York, NY 10009
email: Akashic7@aol.com
website: www.akashicbooks.com

in memory of

Helen Wolfe
&
Ruth Samanowitz

and for my parents

acknowledgments

Thanks to my visionary publisher Johnny Temple and brilliant editor Gabrielle Danchick.

To Elena Georgiou, Marie-Alyce Devieux, Mary McGrail, and Angela Himsel for their passion, creativity, and indispensable support on matters of life and literature. To Debora Lidov for her comments on the manuscript. Also thanks to the following people: Judy Jordan, Claire Holt,Howard Levenson, Lorne Manly, Rebecca Packer, Isabel Pipolo, Jaymie Ridless, J.T. Rogers, Alison Sloan Gaylin, Caryn Stabinsky, and all of the creative souls at my job—the temps shall inherit the earth!

Finally, special thanks to R. D. for two decades of inspiration, collaboration, and treasured friendship.

I hate commonplace heroes and lukewarm emotions, the kind you find in real life.

—Emma Bovary

People's fantasies give them problems. If you didn't have fantasies you wouldn't have problems because you'd just take whatever was there.

—Andy Warhol

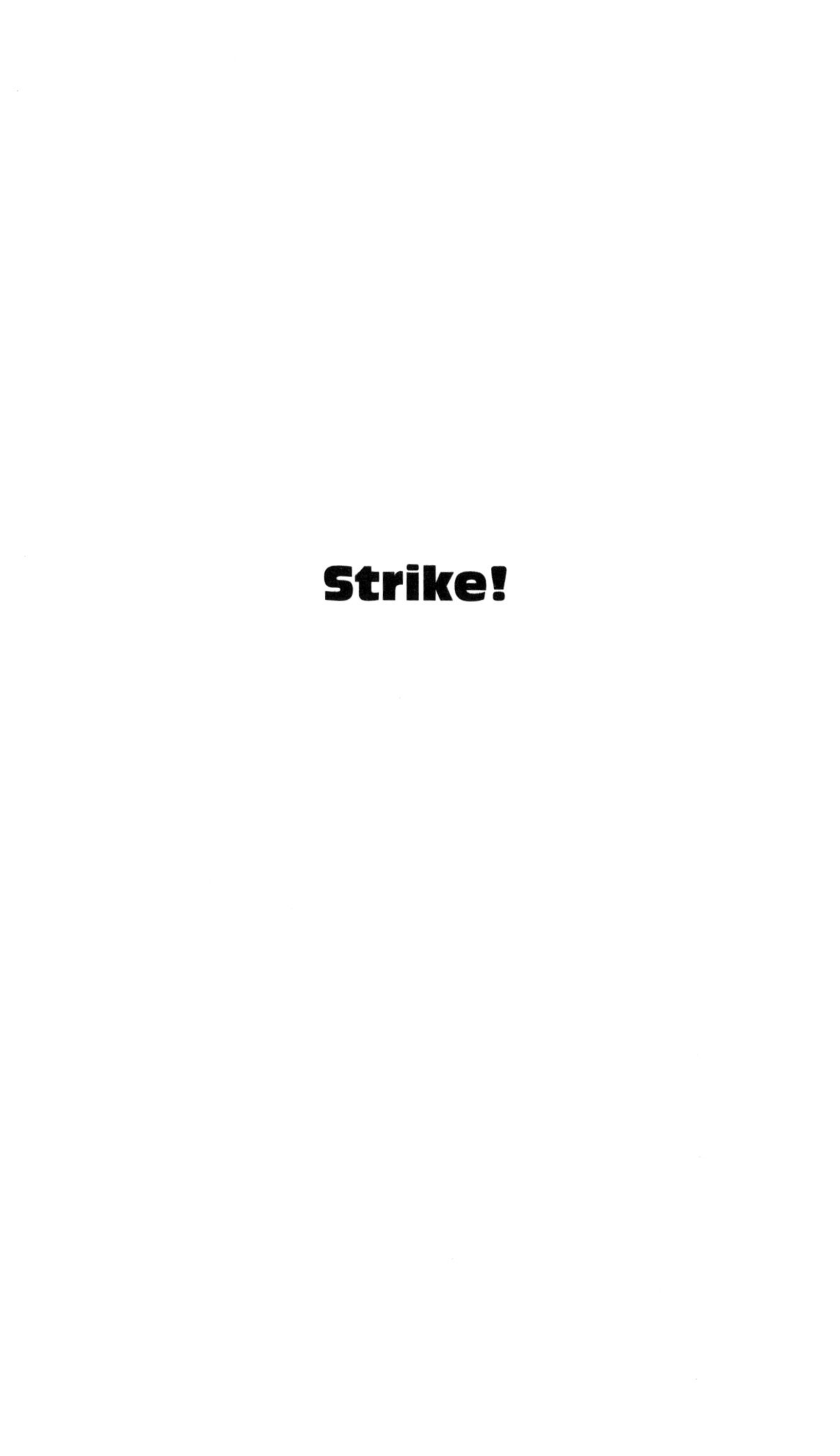

Strike!

Their deaths came on the morning of my thirty-first birthday. It was still dark when I got the call that the double suicide was only minutes away, and that Dr. Milford P. Kaminsky, the self-anointed Master of Self-Deliverance, had secured a simultaneous feed to the local news channel. I'd interviewed Kaminsky a few times since moving back to New York from Miami about a year before to cover the courts for *The City News*, and knew today was what he'd been waiting for: his first televised suicide. A coup if assisted suicide were your genre, your *raison d'etre* so to speak.

I lay in bed watching television with the sound off, as I listened to the waking psalms of New York City: the lackadaisical roar of taxi cabs, the loading and unloading of delivery trucks, garbage trucks, hand trucks; birds chirping like smoke alarms with dying batteries. The primal hour beat a hematite sheen against my window, while inside, the colorless hues of night vision ruled. Everything was smothered in gray. A morose gray, a brooding insinuation. Gray like a worn black-and-white film, but for the rainbow of talking heads on the silent television screen, the flickering red circles on my answering machine and power strip, the green dots from the clock on the VCR. Aggressive mixed messages from the technology department. And so early in the day.

I thought of a fall morning thirty-one years ago when I stepped feet first from Mom's womb: a breecher. She always said it was a bad omen that after properly birthing two boys her daughter had come out ready to leave. She might say I hadn't stopped walking since. If so, I'd strut a huge circle. For I was back home, waiting for my life to take root in this bizarre execution.

The satellite hook-up clicked in and a couple appeared on screen—two humanoid insects with fogged-up plastic bags over their faces. I jolted up to get a better look. Was I dreaming? Hallucinating? I blinked, but there they were, dying on my television screen.

I shut off the mute button and was assaulted by a muffled static. There were no voices, no familiar small-screen sounds. The bodies, one a man and the other a woman, were utterly still. They were holding hands, and behind those smoggy bags their eyes were closed, no longer watching, so I and everyone else watching could stare with impunity at the man's purple veins, the fine white hairs on his knuckles. We could inspect the brownish spots that dotted the woman's hefty arms and read their T-shirts:

I was touched by these two people trying to ensure they would get wherever they were going together and get there in style. What courage to chuckle in death's face, to have one last laugh on life and all of us who'd tuned in to see them off.

My cordless chimed. Before I could say hello, I heard Shade's voice: "Looks like your boy was up early this morning."

"I know, can you believe this? You think it's real?"

"It's on practically every channel."

"But is it live or taped? I mean, how can they stand there filming and not take the bags off? It's obscene."

"Ciao Manhattan! Home of the first septuagenarian snuff film."

"Shush, I want to see the rest," I said, but couldn't stop thinking, *septuagenarian snuff film.* I was jealous I hadn't thought of it myself. A home-girl Dorothy Parker, Shade was queen of the urban mot. Her slick tongue, which had made her quite the astute arts reporter, had always impressed me as well. I had to love her even when I wanted to hate her.

Shade's breath caught when the woman's head plopped over sideways. Then the man's followed, no joke, both heads imitating the arrows on their T-shirts. As sick as I felt I couldn't take my eyes from the TV set.

I'd seen people die on television before: busloads of tourists blown to bits in war-torn countries, cops busting down doors and blasting drug dealers with semiautomatic handguns, public officials pumping lead through their brains. Outright carnage and decimation of entire nations I could stomach over breakfast, but something about these people got to me. They seemed so righteous. And peaceful, too. Even the camera crews held silent vigil until a uniformed police officer arrived and removed the plastic bags from their heads. They were pronounced dead still holding hands.

Then the media converged.

"I'm going to court," I said.

"Yeah? The machinists and drivers went out over the weekend, I bet we're gone by the end of the day."

"I don't care," I said and realized I was pouting. I'd worked long and hard over the last few months to cultivate Kaminsky. The threat of a strike looming at the *News* wasn't enough to stop me. "This is my story," I said.

"Yours and everyone else's now. Pick me up on your way, I can't let you cross the picket line alone."

"I'm not crossing. It's my story, I'll write it for someone else if I have to."

"Not if you want to work in this town. Why do I always feel like I have to protect you?"

"Because you're the one who brought me back here."

"You wouldn't wear sunscreen, a little white girl like you. I had no choice."

Somewhere along the way we'd accepted the truism that Shade had brought me to New York from Miami—where we'd first met working at *The Daily Times*—simply because she'd been the conduit between me and Giordano, the city desk editor here. Convenient of her to forget I'd spent the first twenty-three years of my life in Bay

Ridge, and that my family still lived in the very brownstone I'd grown up in. Handy as well for her to overlook that shortly after I'd rented my studio and had all of my furniture shipped north, *The City News* was sold to a group of belt-tightening, productivity-crazed, vegemite-mad Australians.

But I couldn't blame Shade for the new management team nor its union busting. She knew I'd been looking for a way out of the land of silicon and sunshine.

"I'll be there in an hour."

"Fantastic," she said. "And by the way, Slivowitz, happy birthday."

"Thanks, thanks a lot."

"Just don't forget you're still young enough to be my daughter."

I hung up laughing. Shade was exactly eighteen months older than I was. Even in dog years she probably couldn't have been my mother, but I let her believe she was the older and wiser of us, just as I let her call me Slivowitz. She was one of the few people to whom I'd confessed my name change, after she'd told me why she called herself Shade.

Shade's real name was Teesha Marie Simpson, which she still used professionally. Her parents were doctors who'd pioneered an all-white, upper-middle-class suburb of Atlanta. Shade said she tried to fit in, straightening her hair, smoking pot, and listening to Joni Mitchell albums, but ultimately she felt like a watered-down version of herself. It was the seventies, and in a twisted stance of racial pride, she adopted the name Shade from a blaxploitation film, *Wicked Mamma Jamma,* and stopped answering to the name Teesha.

Her teenage self-possession impressed me, especially since I'd changed my own name from Slivowitz to Silver out of ethnic embarrassment. Back in the old country my father's family had been called Sonnanovicz, but as they emigrated from Poland to Argentina to America and learned to speak English, those who'd made it through Ellis Island thought the name sounded like son-of-a-bitch. So they became Slivowitz, a name still Jewish enough for me to fear it. In my neighborhood some Jewish kid was always getting beaten up or having her skirt lifted by Lotharios-in-training on the way home from Sunday school.

I was saved from going to Sunday school myself. After my brothers bungled their Bar Mitzvahs, Rowdy departing from his prepared speech and talking instead of utopian experiments on Pluto, and Neil a few years later stumbling through one or two lines of transliterated Hebrew before passing out face first on the pulpit, Dad made us quit the temple. "I'm sick of the whole horseshit-ghetto religion anyway," he'd said. With my dark hair and brown eyes, I found I could pass as Italian. My adolescent and teenage years were characterized by the gold, Italian horn necklace I wore, and, whenever I could get away with it, telling people my last name was DeSilva. I'd heard my brother Neil use the name once.

Yet when I marched down to City Hall on my eighteenth birthday, only months after Dad died, it seemed heretical to give up Dad's name for Neil's. Thus followed my rebirth as Rachel Silver. As the years tramped on and I became a journalist, it seemed to make sense. The name looked good in print. I knew it the moment I felt the rush of reading my first byline in the Brooklyn College newspaper; I believed it now as I lay awake in my studio apartment wondering how far I was from being a name out of print.

A surge of fear overtook my body. I rubbed my fingertips against my neck, alarmed by its softness, the loose feel of the skin. Sliding my hands underneath my T-shirt, I felt my breasts, convinced they must have dropped another millimeter since yesterday when I was merely thirty. I'd actually liked turning thirty, was glad to put the scrambling angst of my twenties behind me. Besides, I'd just started working for one of the daily newspapers I'd grown up reading, in the media capital of the world no less.

One year later I was on the verge of unemployment with a body ready to betray me, riding its own course toward the day I might end up on television with a plastic bag over my head. The image puzzled neatly into the visions I'd been having recently, visions of disintegrating piece-by-piece in a Miami nursing home as Grandma had, or like Aunt Lorraine getting bushwhacked by cancer. Then there was my ongoing fear of becoming a wild-haired hermit who lived in a cobwebbed studio with an army of cats and the complete edition of the *Oxford English Dictionary.*

I reached under the covers for Freddy and pulled her to my chest.

I could hold her for maybe three seconds before she started scratching away from me. Some people said it was the operation that made her so prickly—"Really, Rachel, how would you feel if they ripped out your ovaries when you were barely a year old!" But there was another, darker problem with Freddy, the family secret; her parents were brother and sister.

The guy I got her from swore that incest was a sign of royal breeding in animals, though he didn't tell me any of this until I'd already had her a few months. At least she was beautiful: midnight black with white dots like snow falling in bright headlights. I'd called her Moondust until my ex-fiancé Sam said she looked like Fred Flintstone. Thus she was christened Freddy by a man who hated cats. I should have known then I would never marry him and could have avoided the few farcical years to follow. Blame it on my youth, like Chet Baker said. And how I used to play Dad's Chet Baker LPs late into the night, amazed by his voice that mimicked the timbres of his trumpet. With an ear that good, I could only imagine what else he'd heard. Which sort of explains the booze, the pills, the heroin. Which definitely explains why he ended up splattered on the sidewalk in front of his hotel room. Yet, to fly from a window in old Amsterdam had to be more spiritual, more celestial, than ending up the subject of a septuagenarian snuff film on American television.

I got up slowly, sniffling from ragweed air, my muscles sore from a string of sleepless nights. It took all I had just to make it to the bathroom.

Blame it on my youth.... I crooned melodramatically to Freddy, who'd long before wrestled herself from my half-nelson of intimacy and beaten me to the shower. This was one of our best times together, her sitting on the tub in between the shower curtain and liner, me turning the hot water up so high it steamed up the bathroom and made my skin pink. I let the jet stream pummel my spine and shoulders, water dripping down into the small of my back, my ass, in between my thighs, until I felt myself slowly coming alive, huffing against the rhythms of morning.

By the time Shade and I made it downtown, the supreme court

building was a giant octopus, its cupola standing tall above the swaying tentacles of cars and buses and people. Though I resented paying to park, I pulled into the garage next to the family court building to save time.

Shade slipped her cell phone into the pocket of her suede jacket, and its fringes slapped back and forth. She rolled her eyes, "Showtime."

I took a deep breath. We climbed out of my jeep and went off to join the octopus.

I was glad Shade had insisted on coming. She had an enviable way of commanding attention without being ostentatious, of making people believe they'd been waiting just for her. I used to think it had to do with her appearance, the yellow-green eyes and egg-shell brown skin, a combination everyone called "exotic," especially when she braided her hair like a rap diva. But, as I got to know her better, I realized her physicality was merely a promo for the rest of her charms.

Back in Miami, when she had her weekly "Movie Minute" spot on the five o'clock news, strangers used to stop her in restaurants, on the beach, at the Lincoln Road mall. And Shade, whose patience would have made her a good shrink or customer service rep, would talk to everyone, no matter how crazy or disheveled or abusive, though a few in the latter category did force her to whip out a can of pepper spray. To wit: the price of fame. I remember the few times I'd taken her with me to see Grandma at Sunset Estates and all of the Jewish ladies with their personal aides from Trinidad or Haiti went storming the rec room to meet Teesha Marie Simpson. Never mind that I'd just done a four-part series on the home's abuse of Medicare payments, Shade was on television. She was a *celebrity.* She had three names. If ever the imbalance between TV and print had become obvious, it was during those trips to Sunset Estates. Even Grandma was on her best behavior, and only once or twice opened a sentence with the words, "You people." Shade handled it well. "We people," she said. "You mean journalists?"

Shade caught me smiling and said, "What?"

"I was thinking about you and my grandmother."

"I loved that lady."

"She was a racist."

"Listen, my grandmother told me I could spot Jews by the big pores on their noses. Nobody's perfect."

We were climbing the crowded steps of the courthouse, the ones they always flashed in the opening credits of New York City cop shows filmed in Hollywood. The pale gray marble cut a dreary outline against the pale gray clouds, giving an air of soiled ethereality, like an angel trying to quit smoking cigarettes.

Inside, the dark corridors were filled with lawyers, paralegals, secretaries, stenographers, and, of course, the media. Shade and I made our way to the press room, but she lingered in the hallway with another reporter she knew. I headed to the soda machine for a diet Pepsi and the right stake-out point. I needed to see who was there, get a feeling for the buzz before talking to anyone.

Andrew from *The Legal Reporter* was on me immediately. "What are you doing here?" he asked, sounding as concerned as a man with a British accent could.

"Same thing you are."

"But—" He had a worried look I'd seen a lot of recently, mostly from the doctors who diagnosed Aunt Lorraine's cancer. "I'm sorry about the...about your management troubles. The waiting must be unbearable."

"Spare the solidarity. What's up with Kaminsky?"

"I don't know much."

"Come on, out with it or I'll call INS and tell them your marriage is a fraud. Shouldn't some American have your job, anyway?"

He didn't bite. "I really am sorry, Rachel."

"I don't want your job, it was just a joke. Jesus."

Andrew clicked his lips and sighed as if life were too taxing this morning. I knew the feeling. We stared at each other for a second before the tension buckled. He smiled. "Their names were Ida and Marvin Salinger, quite a literary ring don't you think? She had Parkinson's, he was in the early stages of Alzheimer's. They're up to their ears in suicide notes, living wills, the works. Kaminsky, apparently, had them explain everything on video, step-by-step. They took the pills themselves and even tied the little baggies for each other. All so dreadfully legal, I'm assured."

"What about the TV footage? Who shot the footage?"

"As far as we know they rigged the video camera themselves, and my guess is they hit the netherworld long before Kaminsky called the TV people. I'm on line trying to get a copy of the reel. And that, darling, is all she wrote."

"You're a peach, Andrew."

Having come through for me, he excused himself to go and check the dockets.

"Now about your job..." I called after him. He pivoted, blew me a kiss, and then was gone. I hung around asking questions, annoyed by the reaction of my colleagues, some of whom greeted me in cloying sympathy as Andrew had initially, while others ignored me as if I had huge red welts on my skin. That was the toughest bit yet. We always shared information, though I found it best not to believe anything anyone said until I confirmed it myself. You never knew when somebody was trying to fake you out of doing a story or to plant a dud in your laptop. Contrary to popular belief, there were not a million stories in the naked city. You had about three a week. If you weren't floating the few that became water-cooler conversation, you went unnoticed.

I needed Kaminsky. I'd been one of the first reporters to interview him a few months back, and he'd been ecstatic about the coverage. Surely he owed me some kind of exclusive. And with the strike hanging over me, a cumulonimbus ready to burst any second, I needed this story. If I was going down it would be with a bang and not a whimper. I laughed at myself: *You talk a good game in your head, Slivowitz.* When I talked to myself recently I was sounding more and more like Shade.

I left the press room to look for her, figuring I could use her cell to call Kaminsky on his private line. She was standing a few doors down talking to a woman with burgundy hair and a biker jacket. A camera and press pass swung from her neck while she stood, her feet spread and thumbs through her belt loops, as if she were leader of the pack in a Russ Meyer film, and Shade, her sweet prey, leaned her shoulder against the wall, her hips swaying back and forth. Her flirting pose. I'd seen her work it on both women and men—she was bi—but, for some reason, today, I couldn't stomach watching her. A current ran through my body, and I felt claustrophobic.

I hung back until the feeling passed, then decided to interrupt Shade. We were a team: I was transportation, she communication. Damn that woman, I needed the phone. I started walking toward them when Shade caught my eye and met me half-way. Motorcycle Woman fled into a herd of photographers.

"Give me the phone," I said, setting aside all thoughts of her and the woman. "Kaminsky's doing a press conference at three."

"Forget it, Slivowitz, we're out. Tina heard it on her police radio, they sent a fucking flotilla of cops up to the paper."

"Then maybe we should just drive by his office."

"You're not listening." She tugged at my sleeve and looked me straight in the face. "We're on strike. You're not going anywhere. You know what they call people who cross picket lines, don't you?

"Um...employed?"

"Definitely not that."

"Look, you go strike if you want. I'm not into this...this strike thing, these picket lines, any of it. It's bullshit...some driver gets a cramp in his back and we're all supposed to run around like retards carrying placards."

"Watch it, watch it with the tough-girl act."

"Tell me you want to spend the rest of the day screaming hey, hey, ho, ho."

"You have no idea what you're talking about," she said. "It's not like a peace march."

I ran my hand through my hair and looked away. Cliques of media thronging the press room, gray-suited attorneys flocking in and out of the hallway, administrative types wandering outside with unlit cigarettes cupped in their palms...the general life of the courthouse proceeded as usual. It took me back to high school, the cramped corridors, lockers slamming, kids laughing their way into classrooms with tiled floors and dusty windows, as I stood off to the side, watching with institutionalized dread. I hadn't felt this way in a while.

I turned back to Shade, whose lips were pursed to the side and bobbing.

"Stop biting your mouth," I said.

"I can't help it."

"Well, stop. We should go up there, huh?"

She nodded, "I don't think we have a choice."

I threw my bag over my shoulder, and we started walking. "We're not going anywhere without some M&Ms."

"Okay, but I get the green ones."

"You always get the green ones."

We stopped at the candy counter. I searched the colorful packages for a medium-size bag of M&Ms. "What about the blue ones?" I said, paying off the candy man.

Shade raised the corner of her lip. "They're so depressing."

"Depressing?"

"You can have those, I don't even want to deal with blue candy."

We were leaving the candy counter when a woman shouted Shade's name. I knew who it was before she and her burgundy hair made their way over. Shade introduced us. Her name was Tina Macadam, and I immediately thought, phony. Having changed my own name, I suspected the same of everyone else, but *Macadam?* That was like wearing a fake fur or becoming a platinum blonde. Why didn't she just call herself Tina Motorcycle?

Shade told her she couldn't talk now, the strike was calling. "I'll call you," she smiled at Tina Macadam.

"Good, 'cause I'm ready to roll whenever."

"Yeah, it sounds great."

I looked up as if I had important things on my mind while they finished talking about some elusive project and said goodbye. Shade and I were silent on the walk back to my jeep.

"What were you and what's-her-name planning?" I asked as we were buckling up.

"Oh, she's doing a film. She wants me to help write it."

Bullshit, I thought. I didn't trust Tina Macadam around Shade, who was now saying that I, if anyone, should see how a creative project would interest her. A closet fiction writer, Shade had let me see a few stories she'd written, most of which I found too risqué. Who used the word pussy with the frequency of a conjunction? Nevertheless, I sympathized with her yearning for something greater, a passion that would throw her into a deep depression whenever she interviewed a screenwriter or novelist she believed wasn't half as good as she could be if she only had the time. "Our lives are shit," she use to tell me, pluralizing. "We gotta get out of here, everything's so small-time."

"It's Miami, not Chattanooga."

"Not the place, the pattern. I can't stand the thought of spending my life writing about other people who think they're so damn fabulous."

"So quit."

But I knew she wouldn't quit. She suffered from what she called "upper-middle-class paralysis," which, in English, meant her parents had worked their butts off and then spoiled her silly with cars and clothes and cruises while not paying her the least bit of attention. To her family, value was the tangible: a salary, a byline, or, even better, a spot on the local TV news. As for myself, I was the product of an autodidactic electrician who worked sporadic construction jobs and a housewife who before marrying harbored dreams of starring in a Broadway musical, though she was utterly tone deaf. I never understood the tenets of this new-monied anxiety. It seemed to me that Shade, if anyone, could afford to quit her day job. She had rich parents, an IRA, a broker named Butch. A suspicion was borne in me, therefore, that there was more to her existential dilemma than a crisis of materialism.

Perhaps that's why I felt nervous as she spoke about this gig with Tina Macadam, and there was something I didn't like about that woman, an attitude I couldn't quite verbalize, but if I told Shade she would accuse me of being judgmental. As if that were a bad thing.

I downshifted for a red light and found myself saying, "Just be careful."

"Please." She dropped a red, a blue, and a brown M&M into my palm and ate a few green ones. I had to laugh at the determination with which she isolated them, as if she were mining a pile of dirt for diamonds.

"Don't think I didn't see how you looked at her," I said.

"Doesn't matter. I'm through with women."

"Oh you're heterosexual now?"

"No, men too, I'm done with it all," she laughed. I shifted into first as the light changed; then second; and third, moving around a bus with a billboard for men's underwear, thinking how nice it was to be briefly insulated in a little bubble on the streets of Manhattan. If only we could bag the strike and drive around the city all day long eating candy.

Shade had her elbow up against the window, two fingers pressed against her temple in her thinking pose. "Maybe you'll understand this better when you're my age." She raised her eyebrows and I sighed. "Dating is a business negotiation. Everything's an Issue with a capital I, and nobody wants to have fun anymore. It's pathetic, really. Where are the fucking snows of yesteryear?"

"The snows of yesteryear, haven't you heard? They're out on strike."

She smiled. "So it's welcome to the new celibacy."

"Which for me is the same as the old celibacy."

"I don't understand, you're such a catch."

"It's just not that important."

"What?"

"You know, sex, love, whatever."

"I don't believe you."

"It's true," I said, though the real truth was I wasn't very good at any of it. I'd never been in love, moved from one hopelessly inappropriate relationship to the next, and couldn't have an orgasm in the presence of anyone besides Freddy. Men often called me frigid. But how could I explain this to Shade, a woman far less rigid with sex than with her M&Ms?

"Give me a green one, come on," I said.

"All right you can have one, but just one." She turned sideways and leaned her arm over the stick shift. I was busy dodging traffic. "Open."

I did and she dropped the smooth, green pellet on my tongue. I bit down with a loud crunch. "Remember, those things can be dynamite in the wrong hands," she said.

"Who died and made you M&M boss?"

"I was born that way."

"Elitist."

I turned the corner on Forty-second Street, and we were immediately dead-locked in a honking maze of cars, buses, and trucks that even the cyclists and rollerbladers had difficulty cutting through. We sat; we listened to reports of the strike on public radio; we watched the cars pass in the other direction; we moved an inch. Slowly, the stagnating traffic throbbed its way into my brain. I felt as if my head would pop off. "Shit!" I said. "Shit! Shit! Shit!"

"Okay, calm down," Shade said. She had plan B in mind. "Jut out a little bit to the left...that's it, now keep pushing out until you can break into a U-ey."

"Easy for you to say."

"No, look, there's a few feet of opening, go go go!"

"It's a double yellow line—"

"Go!"

I went. Cars honked madly. My heart accelerated, my fingers sweat against the stick shift. Someone called me Jackass. But within a few minutes we were out of traffic. The tingling in my neck settled, though my heart kept its brisk pace. I'd never crossed a double yellow line before. I felt rebellious, nihilistic even. Shade and I couldn't stop smiling, as we headed west toward the second parking garage of the day.

Only when we left the jeep and started walking toward the picket line did it hit me that this strike could get expensive. Very expensive, indeed.

Unlike the molluscan mass outside the courthouse, the crowd gathered in front of *The City News* formed an amorphous and angry blob swallowing anything in its wake. I stayed along the outskirts of the police barriers, while Shade adapted more quickly to the scene. Someone handed her a placard, and I lost her to the sea of black jackets, television cameras, and receding hairlines, until she returned and dragged me kicking and screaming to the center of the crowd where a few other reporters had staked out turf next to a hot dog stand.

I was uncomfortable with the spectacle of these heretofore mild-mannered, Clark Kent and Lois Lane reporters morphing seamlessly into fiery Bolsheviks. There were James, the Asian mensch as Shade called him, raising his fist in the air, and Carrie, the twitchy City Hall reporter who always wore business suits, wielding a placard that said: Union Rights = Human Rights. They had to know how ridiculous they looked. The whole scene was as absurd as a song and dance number from the Broadway musicals my mother revered. Even Shade was screaming loud enough that her voice became Lauren Bacall husky. Slowly, however, amid all of the shouting and sloganeering, a strange energy overwhelmed me, and I wondered whether I was the one who appeared ridiculous among the frenzied ralliers. Testing myself, I took a step forward, raised my fist and shouted: "Back off union busters!" My cheeks flushed, but nobody seemed to notice. I was just another voice in the crowd. A few more chants and I felt invigorated, unraveled, as if my life had a discernible purpose, if only temporarily. Soon, I was cheering along as strikers threw bottles at armored delivery trucks and chided any mutt who crossed the line. I became indignant when reporters from the other dailies, gathering material for tomorrow's papers, descended upon us. Was frozen as photographers snapped our pictures.

Later, other unions joined a solidarity rally. Thousands of people gathered around us, the nucleus, chanting, carrying signs, even hurling a few cans or old newspapers. The smell of sauerkraut stained the air.

At once, we'd become part of history, descendants of the Boston Tea Party, brothers and sisters to the Pullman Strikers, United Auto Workers, and Air Traffic Controllers. We were the working-class darlings of the moment, which, after a while, made me nervous. For we in the media should know better than anyone how quickly the moment comes and goes. Tomorrow, as the fringes of this angry mob reported for work, we would remain in the streets alone.

I broke from the cacophony and leaned back against a grimy, brick office building. Looking westward I spotted the sky, a magical cast of blue peeping in between the buildings as if the atmosphere itself had been artificially manufactured, pink and blue as far as my eye could see. This was the sky I'd imagined in those junior high science classes when I first tripped the magic of acids and bases, the sky I'd even earlier taken it upon myself to draw with a rainbow of Crayolas.

"Moron girl!" Rowdy had said. "There ain't no pink clouds."

"There are," I tried to explain, recalling something Dad had read to me from the encyclopedia about the sun's rays being refracted, which I'd heard as reefer-acted, like the reefer Rowdy and Neil smoked. There was smoke and there was light and it all came from the sun.

"When the sun moves," I said, "it paints the clouds different colors, it makes them pink."

"Pink like your cunt," Neil said, barreling into the living room with his tongue wiggling around his lips. "Pink to red and then you're a bloody-cunted bitch for the rest of your life." He put his face close to mine and whispered, "Blood cunt, blood cunt. . . ."

I ran upstairs to my bedroom, locked the door behind me and waited for the pounding to stop. When I got my period a few years later, I knew that Neil had foretold it. By then he'd started his watching, too. I couldn't insert a tampon or take a shit in the house without feeling his eyes on me. Even though Neil was gone now, living in Las Vegas, he was probably still drilling holes in some wall or door to scope out other unsuspecting women. I was as certain of this as I was then of those pink clouds in Brooklyn.

We congregated across the street at The Corral to see the strike unfold as the rest of the world would see it, but soon found the top spot on every six o'clock broadcast devoted to Kaminsky and his dead protégés. Our fifteen minutes arrived after the Kaminsky story. Tony ordered pitchers of margaritas and tequila shots for everyone.

"Look look, there I am!" Michael said, pointing to his face on the three television screens behind the bar.

"You look like a longshoreman," Tony said. "That's why they used you."

It was true. Some of us may dress like lawyers or talk like street-corner philosophers or eat in trendy restaurants, but when the line is drawn, reporters fall on the side of labor. Working class was the look the TV cameras were going for.

"Turn it up, I want to hear my sound bite," Michael said.

The curmudgeonly bartender obliged. He'd been working at The Corral long enough to know that a strike meant increased business.

"Oh man they cut it," Michael said. "They cut the part where I said seeing all of you run out to the picket line was like watching people march to the gallows."

"That was too literary, too dramatic," I said.

"Just you wait. Try Channel Seven, let's see if superstar Kim Mathews gets all weepy."

"There was some survey recently," Shade said, "I don't remember where, but eight out of ten Americans said they would rather have dinner with Kim Mathews than the President."

"Seems reasonable," Tony said and nobody argued.

The bartender surfed the channels, but kept coming up with the same old story told through the same somber eyes of our TV brethren. There were the management spokesmodels spouting about generations of padded wage and benefit contracts that had made the paper a money pit; the union leaders swearing they would cripple the paper and force the Aussies out of town; and a few comments from strikers, mostly reporters, and, within that subgroup, mostly Michael. Who knew he was such a publicity whore?

As stories of the strike tapered off, the bartender turned down the sound on the TV sets in favor of classic rock: The Doors. A table opened up, and we grabbed it. Tony ordered more shots. "What should we drink to?" he said.

"Let's drink to the dead couple," Michael said. "What were their names?"

"Ida and Marvin Salinger," I said.

"Here's to Ida and Marvin."

"Cheers."

Etcetera. Etcetera. Etcetera.

Everyone drank again—except for me. I'd already had two shots and couldn't risk another. I hated getting drunk, though I'd learned not to make a big deal about it. If I had to I could quickly dump a shot on the floor, cover the glass with my whole hand and pop it back against my mouth while pretending to swallow. It worked every time.

"We need more margaritas," Tony said.

"Don't they come in any other color?" Shade asked, and the next time they came back blue. She grimaced. Eyeing each other across the table, I remembered the blue M&Ms. I'd never known anybody so affected by primary colors.

The drinks kept coming, but we were tired of drinking to Ida and Marvin. "Anybody got a paper?" Michael said. "Get the obits. We'll drink to every goddamn dead person in there."

Shade hurled a copy of *The City News* at him.

"This is getting sick," Carrie said, wobbling up out of her seat. "Doesn't it bother any of you that this morning two people were alive and because of some modern Joseph Mengele tonight they're...." She shook her head back and forth.

"Aw, come on now, sit down," Tony said. "We're just goofing. If we started taking this shit too seriously we'd all be running for the cyanide."

"I know, I know." She took a deep breath and smoothed out her skirt as if she'd learned it in some dress-for-success seminar. Rule #9: Straight Clothing = Straight Thinking. "Look, it's been a monster day, I'm calling it quits." She picked up her briefcase and swung her blazer over her arm. "See you guys," she said.

We said goodbye and then fell silent, as if Carrie's disappearance might force us to address our presence at The Corral. I could hear Jim Morrison's trippy baritone being eclipsed by the clanking bottles and background chatter.

"What's up with Carrie?" Michael said.

"Gee, I don't know," I said.

"Don't you start flipping out now," Tony said.

"Give her a break," Shade said. "She was following Kaminsky."

"Poor Rachey," Tony reached over and patted my head.

"I was just getting comfortable here," I smiled and let him put his arm around me. "And this was so easy, a tailor-made, front-page extravaganza. Shit."

"Yeah, missing out on the story of the century must suck holy rat cock," Tony said.

"It's bigger than a rat, Dibenedetto," I took his arm from my shoulder and stood up.

"Oh nice, asshole, you scared her off, too," Michael said.

"Mind your business, sound-bite boy," Tony said. Then, running his thumb and forefinger against his mustache, he looked up at me. "Come on, I'm sorry, you can come back."

"Relax, I'm just getting a soda."

I had to break away from them, if only to drop the tough-girl act for a few minutes. At the bar, I ordered a diet Coke and bummed a cigarette from the bartender. Though I'd quit a few years ago, smoking was an ongoing battle. These days my resolve was to not buy them, but the way I felt when I took that first drag, as if the smoke going inside helped make sense of everything happening outside, was similar to Carrie smoothing down the wrinkles on her skirt. I took a deep drag, thinking, cancer sticks. Aunt Lorraine had never smoked a day in her life and she got it; genetics weren't on my side.

I put out the cigarette after a few drags and on my way back to the table bumped into James. He was wearing his coat and, like me, seemed a bit awkward amid the streams of tequila shots and smoke and rock-and-roll.

"Strange day," he said.

"It's my birthday."

"Thirty?"

"Plus one."

"I don't know what to tell you."

"Nobody does. Leaving?"

"Yeah, I have to get back to Jersey, I want to put my kids to bed." He pulled the belt of his tan raincoat and smiled. Shade was right about the Asian mensch thing. James was a good guy, and though only thirty-four himself, he seemed much older than the rest of us. Maybe it was the raincoat.

"Take care of yourself, okay?" he said.

"Yeah, you too."

I watched him walk out, then scavenged another cigarette before returning to the table.

We stayed out late. Very late.

I didn't know about anybody else, but I couldn't face the thought of going home to my solitary crib. As people scattered away, Shade and I gravitated to a table full of bundlers who all seemed to be named Bill. She was drunk; I'd been faking it for the last couple of hours. I stayed quiet, turned down drinks when the Bills offered despite Shade's exasperated stares. The feeling I'd experienced earlier with Tina Macadam returned, only now I was skeptical of Shade. For someone who'd just this afternoon joined the ranks of the newly celibate, she was acting quite flirtatious. All of the Bills wanted to take her home.

She was having none of that, however. I could tell by the way she clung to my arm as we finally left the bar and entered the cool, damp night. More than once here in New York I'd seen her work the persiflage, smiling wide-eyed for the boys, and then use me as her foil. She was more talk than action, but I was neither.

We took a taxi back to my jeep, and I drove Shade to her apartment. Before climbing out, she leaned closer to me and smiled. "You're a good kid, Sliver-Twit," she said, spinning a dipsomaniacal derivation of the name that was no longer my own.

"Thanks," I said. I didn't know what else to say and the way she looked at me sometimes, the way she was looking at me now, made any words at all seem redundant. She leaned over and kissed me on the cheek. The next thing I knew the passenger door slammed shut. I watched her climb the steps of her brownstone and disappear behind two sets of glass doors.

Orifice Politics

I ended the first week of the strike at the dentist's office. Camille the dental assistant propped open my mouth and slipped the slurpy, suckling tube beneath my tongue. Water laced with mouthwash showered into the plastic cup. The hairs on my arms stood in collective shiver as Camille hummed to "Top of the World" by the Carpenters.

"She'll be in in a minute," Camille said, trying her best at comfort before Dr. Janis started her drilling. I sat back and wondered why I'd kept this appointment, how my first trip outside since the strike began had me choking the metal beads of the spit-bib.

The last few days had been a fog of frozen pizza and six packs of diet root beer, monotonous words springing from my television set. Only when armed with the channel clicker was I safe from the mocking jeers of my laptop and microcassette, the ridicule of my barren reporter's notebooks. The tools of my trade had given me structure, now all I had was television. And I gave over willingly, letting in the call-in shows and sci-fi sitcoms, the Spanish Harlem hit parade, microorganism hour, *Le Soufflé.* Shows blended into each other; like a pure-bred zombie, I formulated interactive character plots, tracked stray Cheerios from channel to channel. I forgot to feed Freddy until she dug her nails into my arm and drew blood. We started smelling like the litter box.

Then there was the onslaught of phone calls from Aunt Lorraine beginning on the morning after the double suicide, waking me at seven when I'd been out so late the night before. "So that's your Doctor Kaminsky?" she asked. "Why didn't you tell me?"

"He's not my doctor," I assured her. Though I was tired, the way she said *your* kept me alert. It was the tone she used when Mom was badgering her, and I would have to interfere, because like it or not, Mom was *mine.* Just as she was Aunt Lorraine's sister-in-law. But I had no such claim on the suicide doctor. I couldn't even speak of him and Aunt Lorraine in the same breath, let alone imagine bringing them together for a cup of coffee.

Besides, how bad could her cancer be if she was calling me a few times a day. There was such verve in her voice. "I just want to talk to him," she said.

"You have plenty of people to talk to."

"Who, your mother? Rowdy? You tell me, who? Everyone's so tip-toe, hush-hush, and get out. Nobody says anything."

"What do you want from them?"

"I don't know, I just need to talk to somebody...somebody who understands. I'm dying, you know."

"No you're not."

"Say it if it makes you feel better, but you have no idea." I don't know if saying it made me feel any better, but it did help to dull the impact of her words. At least until the next phone call. The problem was we had such easy access to the phone; each of us confined to bed with everything around us grinding to a halt. By the time Camille called reminding me of my appointment with warnings about not filling cavities at this stage—the adult mouth being a bottomless pit of foreign matter, its lacunae home to more toxic garbage than a Staten Island dump—I could hardly refuse an opportunity to shower, dress, and leave my apartment.

Camille, still singing to the Carpenters *(not a cloud in the sky, got the sun in my eye),* clicked her heels against the floor in time. I was so focused on her routine I didn't notice Dr. Janis coming in until she was standing over me, rapacious blond mane swallowing the shoulders of her freshly pressed lab coat. She smelled like she'd just come in from the street. In her hand was the shiny, silver Novocain gun.

"You don't really need it," she said.

"Oh, yech, I do."

The needle bit into my outer gum area no worse than Freddy would do. I cringed, turned my head slightly, and saw Dr. Janis's shoes—cherry combat boots. I trusted her.

Within a few minutes my throat felt numb. Dr. Janis snapped a rubber glove over each of her hands, and I thought of this reporter I used to work with who mangled clichés. She once told me the problem with men—and this goes back to the mid-eighties—was they were becoming too sensitive. "It's like you have to treat them with rubber gloves," she said. At the time I found her stupidity hilarious, although now, I wondered whether she might have been on to something about handling life with latex.

Dr. Janis pulled down my lower lip with a rubber-coated pinkie. As she reached for the drill, I felt the muscles in my stomach contract.

"Relax," she said. "It won't be that bad."

I raised my eyebrows.

"Remember your abscess?" Dr. Janis leaned forward. I could hear the piercing whir of the drill. "You thought you were going to die, remember?"

"Ich was...grosch."

"But you lived to tell."

I nodded affirmatively. I lived. Aunt Lorraine was dying. I imagined her sitting in a chair like this, only instead of Novocain the gun pumped liquefied Seconal, Nembutal, or whatever hemlock of the moment. Dying should not be like going to the dentist. It would have to be less stressful.

"You're so jittery today," Dr. Janis said. "It's just a couple of cavities."

"I told you, she's on strike," Camille interjected.

"Oh, right, right. So what do you do now?"

I shrugged.

"Hey, we have that guy, maybe she can write for him," Camille said, her short, Betty Boop curls bouncing into my peripheral view. "You know, Phillip, the one who does those farm magazines."

"The *Weekly Cow.*"

"No, it's *Cow Week.*"

"And what's the other one? My favorite."

"He's got like tons."

"*Suburban Hog,* that's the one I'm thinking of," Dr. Janis said, nursing a subtle sparkle in her eyes. "They're big in Texas."

"Huge in Texas," Camille said. She and Dr. Janis smiled at each other.

"I don't think Rachel wants to write about farm animals," Dr. Janis said. "You don't, right?"

I gave as much of a grimace as I could manage given that my mouth was propped open by Dr. Janis' hand. I could smell my saliva on her gloves and was feeling too much pressure from the drill against my jaw. Lest my tongue lunge to stop it, I pointed to my mouth and said what surfaced as: "*Uh-gunk-kah.*"

"More Novocain?"

I nodded, and she slipped the metal gun between her thumb and forefinger. This time I couldn't feel the needle.

Lying back supine, legs propped up in the rigor mortis of the moment with Dr. Janis drilling deep into the estuaries of my enamel, I couldn't escape the carnality of modern dentistry. I wondered how Dr. Janis dealt with it. I once asked my ex-fiancé Sam, the gynecologist-in-training, how he could look inside vaginas every day and divorce himself from the notion of sex. "Oh grow up, Rachel," he sneered. Some pussy doctor he turned out to be. But by then sex had become our Issue with a capital I, as Shade would say, and we'd made it into counseling, a dehumanizing experience if ever there was one. I hated the therapist, the way she prodded and probed, with Sam sitting there oafishly, convinced she could shed light on our "problem": my inability to achieve orgasm with him. With anyone.

Because I could come alone, if I concentrated hard enough, masturbation had always seemed a miscarriage of the act itself. Like the now-taunting gaze of my impotent microcassette and laptop, my solitary orgasms reminded me of what I could not otherwise do. Echoed the psychological peanut gallery (in accents of dreary German no less): *But are you sexually frrrrus-tra-ted?* Of course I was sexually frustrated, but I didn't normally have time to think about it, just as I didn't normally have time to deal with cavities.

"You're getting a little mushy above the bicuspid area," Dr. Janis said after she'd finished drilling. She suggested I use a soft-bristle brush as we walked together to the front desk. "Take a couple of Advils if you feel any pounding," she said.

I nodded, my jaw liquid as a Salvador Dali clock. Camille ran my American Express card through the computer.

"And call us if you want to talk to Phillip," she said.

I looked up. "Phillip?"

"The cow guy."

"Oh sure, thanks," I nodded, thinking, over my unemployed body. *Cow Week?* I'd rather stay in bed all day eating frozen pizza straight from the box.

Camille handed me my credit card, and I was then let loose onto the crowded streets of midtown Manhattan on this too-sunny October day. Off to the picket line with the residue of Novocain palsying a side of my face.

At home, my answering machine blinked a torpid two. I paced, listening to the tape scuttle back to the weary iambs of Aunt Lorraine's voice: "Your Doctor Kaminsky was just on again. He is such a spunky fellow, and so good at his—" I jammed my finger on the fast-forwarded button. If only repression could always be this easy.

There was another message; Ethan confirming dinner tonight. I'd canceled our last two appointments as I did often with ex-boyfriends of the married variety who after one drink became sloppy and nostalgic about how great the two of us would have been together now that he was conveniently affixed to somebody else. All right, this only happened with Ethan. But he did say he might have work for me, maybe a celebrity-stroking piece for the glossy fanzine he edited. I heard some of his writers were swimming in cash, and Ethan himself had all of the trappings of financial success—the TriBeCa loft and summer house in the Hamptons, the fast car and bland bandshell of a wife.

Cordless pressed against my ear, I walked to the window, but instead of Ethan I called Shade. Dusk skipped down the street in a dervish of blues that sent the bright orange sun sinking into the Hudson. Cars honked, a child cried for her mother, and Shade wasn't home.

Trading the phone for a pair of 7 x 50 World War II binoculars I found a few weeks ago at a flea market, I spied people walking down Broadway, jackets tossed over their shoulders, some wheeling babies in strollers, others carrying flowers in paper wrapping. Sentimental fools lapping up these last stolen moments of summer. I wanted someone to get hit by a bus.

And where was Ms. Teesha Marie Simpson on this evening oh-so-balmy? Off somewhere with Tina Motorcycle, no doubt. I tried to imagine it...Shade sitting in a dark bar, tilting her head back and laughing, her mouth open so wide you could see the silver fillings on her bottom molars—I loved that, the way she laughed as if nothing had ever felt so good. I thought about ringing her cell phone, but then I might appear too interested in her whereabouts, or simply psychotic, when she picked up and I didn't have a single thing to tell her. I often worried about people thinking I was crazy.

Instead, I called Ethan and said yes, we were still on.

We met at a little bistro near his office. I ate a grilled chicken salad and drank two glasses of wine through our standard punctilio: small talk of careers—or lack thereof in my case, though I was careful not to seem too desperate for work—and friends we had in common from journalism school. After dinner we took the elevator to the top of the Empire State Building and pushed our noses into the grooves of the tall, metal fences, looking down on the lighted buildings of Manhattan as the sticky breezes blew Tropic-of-Cancer waves beneath the bucketing sky. I was feeling a little tipsy, Ethan said he was sober. I got vertigo, he didn't. I practically fell into his arms up there on top of the world, and, though it seemed as sappy as Camille the dental assistant singing the Carpenters, I let Ethan take me home.

Blame the makeshift romance, blame the wine. Or blame it on Shade as I would the next day, but that night I was to break my sixteen months and three weeks—give or take a few days—of celibacy.

It wasn't the sex I'd missed, it was that I was beginning to forget my own body. I needed to be touched. And Ethan was there.

I liked kissing him more than I remembered. He'd become aggressive, his tongue running along the surface of my gums, his lips sucking mine as if through me he could finally breathe.

Soon enough, our clothes were flying overhead, and we were naked with his head planted between my legs, for a long, long time. Ethan was not one to give up easily—this I remembered. But what first felt good soon turned cold and my mind started wandering...don't forget to call Aunt Lorraine...and where was Shade, goddammit?...I wanted a cigarette, but would have to hit the deli on the corner and buy a pack of Marlboros, no, something lighter, if I was going to buy a pack....This was pathetic. Woody Allen had done so many of these scenes it was hard not to imagine myself a split-screen vision, and with Ethan going at it like a lawnmower. It was a shame, because one of the things about being with someone you haven't been with in a few years is you want to show them how much you've improved and on that score I hadn't made much progress. I thought about throwing in an *oooh* here, an *aaah* there, but couldn't. Beyond comprehension was the fact that I often faked being drunk, pretended more than once to be a lawyer to get my hands on legal documents, frequently lied my way into interviews, yet I couldn't fudge an orgasm! This had to stop. I grabbed Ethan's hair and lifted up his head, which for all I knew he'd mistaken as my climax. Then again, he would know better. But he was breathing canine-hot like the weather, and I was just ready to be done with it.

He tore open a condom package, rolled over his dick with latex smelling like the gloves that earlier had covered Dr. Janis' fingers, and I climbed on top of him, rocking him hard and fast enough that I thought I might have felt something myself, if I had anything left of myself to feel. "Slow down," he said and I went faster, almost amused that I could have this penis diving mechanically in and out of my body and not feel a goddamn thing. My vagina was on Novocain, making me tense, hyperaware of the action, yet unable to register any sensation. But I *had* to feel something, so I swung violently up and down ignoring Ethan when he said, "It's too much, I'm going to come," and instead kept up my pace as we went back and forth, him huffing, "I'm going to come," and me heaving, "Come," until he said he didn't want to come, not yet, because it had been so long, and I said not as long as it was for me, and we were suddenly having a conversation in the middle of our thrusts, which made me angry, and wishing I had weight enough to crush him, I slammed my body down on top of him, and he screamed, "Fran's pregnant!" The room went quiet. I looked down at his red face...his black hair...his white teeth...black and white and red all over, like a cow in a blender...fucking *Cow Week!* I laughed maniacally, but only for a breath or two, until I felt a sharp pain pound up into me, and I didn't know whether to scream or be thankful that I finally felt something when another jolt came up through my chest, and then another and another until Ethan screamed "Oh god fuck!" and I wanted to smack the surly look from his face, but instead fell forward on top of him, slid my head against the thin, wet hairs on his chest, and listened to the beat of his heart retreat before raising my head and staring down at the little man-boy soon to be somebody's father. I wanted to puke.

I rolled over on my back and covered my eyes with my elbow. "You can go now," I said.

"Come on, don't do this."

"No, don't talk. Just go."

I kept my eyes covered, listening to the sounds of Ethan dressing, the swish of his zipper, the clink of his belt buckle, every sound amplified as if with his clothing he could smite the heavy silence that hung between us. Then I had to look up and catch his sullen stare as he put on his shoes.

Freddy strolled up and lay languorously at his feet with her arms and legs outstretched. She was such a little tease, reminded me of Shade actually. Ethan couldn't resist and went to pet her. She clamped down on his finger.

"Ow!" He lifted his hand as if he might hit her.

"Touch her and I'll kill you."

He shook his head. "You know, you haven't changed at all. You just sit there all cold like a—I don't know, like a statue. Everything's so tied up in your convoluted perceptions of power."

"My convoluted what! You mention your pregnant wife when

you're about to...you know, whatever." I tried running my fingers through my hair, but was halted by clumps of dry mousse. I squeezed my fists until my scalp burned.

"Come, the word is come. You still can't say it."

"Would you just go home! We'll call it a mistake and walk away."

"You did that already, know what I'm saying? There's no airplane this time."

"No, just wives and babies, what was I thinking?" I sat defiantly. Counted backwards from ten, waiting for him to be gone, but he stayed there staring at me. I folded my arms over my knees, the red sheet tenting in between them, then leaned forward, taking a deep, long breath. "Jesus, Ethan, what are we doing?"

He shook his head back and forth, his eyes softening into contrition, his palms and mouth agape. "I don't know," he said finally, and we mirrored each other with monkey-see-monkey-do gestures until the whole thing seemed so damn absurd.

He walked to the front door. I followed. He turned and looked at me with his silk blazer draped over his shoulders. If I could have named the designer his latest collection probably filled the pages of *Jammin'*. Ethan was never much for integrity, nor journalism. The glorified gonzo life suited him well.

"So, I guess I'll see you," he said.

"Yeah, sure."

He leaned over and kissed the top of my head. I looked up, smiling slightly, wishing he would just leave, because with every lingering second I grew colder, petrified like stone, or what did he call me? A statue.

After he left I remained numb. Riding an insomniac's rage, I scrutinized the sheets for any sign of him—a smell, a stain, a leftover pubic hair—something to prove he was actually here and qualify the emptiness I felt, just as I used to search my bed for quarters left by the tooth fairy, a small compensation for the gaping hole between my teeth. Once, sleeping with my head above a tooth, I felt Neil's hands underneath my pillow. I screamed. Dad came in and they fought violently, punching and grabbing at each other like amateur boxers. They were both red in the face when Dad, finally, using all of his weight, took down his pubescent son.

"You steal quarters from your sister!" Dad screamed.

"Fuck off," Neil said, and they eyed each other so viciously I wanted to bury my head in my pillow.

Dad let go of Neil's arms and stood up.

"Drunk loser ass," Neil mumbled, and, despite Dad's fingerprints all over his neck, he towered out of the room as if he'd been victorious. Dad slammed the door behind him and tucked me back into bed. Still wearing his Milky Way brown leather jacket and smelling of cigarettes and onions, he sat down next to me with his tan boots hanging over the edge of my bed. Just to make sure Neil couldn't take anything else. He stayed sentry until the sun came up. I know, because I woke to him silently slipping away.

I bounded up when the phone rang, knowing immediately who it was. "Were you sleeping?" Aunt Lorraine said as I lifted the receiver.

"It's two-thirty in the morning."

"You don't know what's going on here," she said. "Rowdy won't wash dishes or shower, the government's talking to him through the water or something, I don't know. Everyone's crazy—really! I can't trust them anymore. Your mother said she'd take the phone away."

"Okay, calm down. Nobody's taking your phone away. I'll talk to Mom."

"Her, I don't care. She's worse than those doctors, treating me like I'm some kind of baby, but I know exactly what's going on."

I got out of bed and walked over to the kitchenette. "What do you want?" I asked, turning on the floor lamp next to the counter. My eyes adjusted to the muddy light.

"You know what I want, your—"

"No you don't."

"I do!" Her voice stopped me cold it was so childlike.

"Look, he probably won't even take my calls. I'm no use to him anymore." I heard my tone growing harsh, felt the back of my neck get all hot and sweaty. I was still suffering from the remnants of a lousy lay. And I didn't have a job. And now Aunt Lorraine was deserting me.

Worse, I was sick of playing death's little emissary in this family. It began the day Dad dropped dead of a heart attack, and Mom, who'd been seeing shrinks for as long as I can remember, finally graduated to the psycho clinic. She showed up at the funeral two days later looking like Gloria Swanson in big sunglasses, flanked by two extraordinarily beautiful nurses. Sobbing through the rabbi's soliloquy, she fell to the ground before the service was over. We all ran to her, but the nurses stopped us, one handling crowd control, the other reaching into her pocket for smelling salt. Mom rose dramatically, smiling beyond those of us who'd gathered around her as if the footlights rendered us invisible. The nurses led her out and that was the end of Dad's funeral.

Aunt Lorraine was more Bette Davis in *All About Eve.* She believed drama was better left to the stage or at least confined behind locked doors. Then why the urge to see Kaminsky? He was all image, nothing but a spin-doctored psychopomp.

"Honey, I just want to talk to him," she pleaded with me. I stood silently at the kitchen counter, naked underneath my red sheet.

"I heard he's from Poland," she said. "Both of his parents were killed in Auschwitz. We're practically related."

"Then why don't you call him?" I lifted my left pinkie to my teeth and gnawed.

"How can you say that? You have no idea how I feel, you barely know what you feel. You're such a journalist sometimes."

"Not anymore. I'm nothing now."

"Stop feeling sorry for yourself. I'm dying and don't you try and tell me anything different, because I'm sick of taking care of everyone else's troubles. I need you, you understand?"

I took a deep breath, picked at my chapped lips with my fingernails. I couldn't stay mad at her for getting sick, for seeking out even the most bizarre anesthesia. "All right, I'll call him," I said finally. "But just to talk."

"That-a-girl," she said.

When we hung up I was in the bathroom. I lifted my red toga and peed, hoping the warm liquid might thaw out my vagina, yet I felt nothing but a vain hole between my legs. I might as well be Barbie.

Standing up, I caught a quick glance in the mirror. My eyes burned into my face, the eyes of death's messenger, unemployed adulterer and feckless father-fucker. I hated myself, but looked striking. I could be beautiful even, my eyes blacker than black and feral, my face spirited with anger. For the first time in a while I wanted to masturbate.

The next day it rained.

Outside, pellets bounced from the pavement; inside, windows fogged against the dreary, wet day. Shade and I sat across from each other at our half-way point, an art deco café on Ninth Avenue in the upper Forties called The Movie House.

I curled my fingers around my big gulp latté, bending my head down so the steam came wafting up my nose. Good for the allergies.

"Rain, schmain," Shade said. She sipped her orange mocha frappé through a straw.

"It's funny, I can't remember rain in Miami."

"What are you talking about? It was always raining. Remember the hurricane? We had to evacuate your grandmother."

"Sure, hurricanes, but regular rain?"

She leaned her arm on the empty chair next to her and smiled. "How about after the Redford preview when we got stuck on Joey's boat?"

"Oh my god. We had to sit in that cabin watching his one music video over and over and over."

"Hey, he had a vision," she pursed her lips.

"Please...and Sam kept calling him Johnny."

We smiled in recognition. Shade's boyfriends, sporadic though they were, tended to be souped-up con men—usually in advertising or the music business—who made Sam feel inferior for wanting to do something as unglamorous as perform pelvic exams and diagnose yeast infections. I had to admit I got off on Sam's inferiority complex. With him, I actually experienced myself as having the cool life, just as with Shade I felt as if my life were not cool enough.

Shade used to namedrop the crazy people she knew, the wild

places she frequented, and she'd cloaked an air of mysteriousness around the women she dated. So adept she'd been at velvet roping the disparate parts of her life. Now, she was out and proud. Maybe it was a New York thing, but in the year I'd been back I'd already met three different girlfriends, not including Tina Macadam. Apparently, they'd had what Shade said was an uneventful date last night, which I knew meant that Shade didn't have sex, as opposed to my own nonevent.

I brought my latté to my lips and inhaled a dollop of foam. "Can I ask you a question?"

"Sure."

My heart sped up involuntarily. I unzipped my sweater, but kept it hanging from my shoulders. "Why didn't you? Last night?"

"With Tina?"

"Is there someone else?" I asked, terrified she might say yes. My reaction shocked me, that it suddenly mattered so much.

"No, no," she nodded. "There's no one else."

I was relieved and couldn't help smiling. She smiled back. Before I knew it, we were deep gazing, and I was taken back to those times in Miami when she told me about her sex life, and I remembered being jealous that she had a sex life, while Sam and I were engaged in a tiresome psychological battle over my orgasms. It occurred to me now that my jealousy might have been misplaced.

Her brow furrowed as if she were thinking big. "You know how they say be careful what you want because you might get it?" I nodded blindly, unable to stop staring at her. "Well, let's just say I'm trying to be careful."

"She wouldn't sleep with you, huh?"

"You little bitch," she smiled. "I'll have you know it was the other way around, actually. I find I'm getting more prudish with age." She leaned her elbows on the table, crossed her arms over her breasts with a slight tilting forward of the shoulders. Her eyes telegraphed a catch-me-if-you-can quality. I could see how she attracted both men and women. But screw the rest of them. She was getting to me.

I felt as if I were entering the shallow end of a swimming pool, adjusting step by step to the cold water. The thing is, I never learned how to swim. You don't in Brooklyn.

Shade rolled her lipstick-stained straw in between her fingers amid the simmering hum of the café. I had to sit on my hands to keep them from shaking.

"And you?" she said. "What ever possessed you to go to bed with Ethan again?"

I wanted to say, You, you idiot. You, because I called you first and you weren't there; you, because I was jealous of you and Tina; you, because I was feeling rejected and needed comfort. But I didn't get anything close to it. Oh, what I would have given to utter half of what I was thinking, if only I understood it myself. Instead, I remained impenetrable: a frizzy-haired wall.

"It was just one of those things," I said.

"One of those things. Yeah, right." She pursed her lips.

"I'm serious."

"You don't have sex for months and end up with Ethan, he's a total dog. There's something else, what aren't you telling me?" She stared at me with her spicy mustard eyes, so I stared back, tongue-tied. Rain slapped and streamed next to us, giving cinematic pause as we lapsed into stone.

Shade shifted in her seat without taking her eyes away from me. "Come on, what is it?" she said.

"He said he might have work, all right?" My pulse jolted at the iciness of my tone. Actually, Ethan had left a message earlier telling me he had a job for me, but I felt too creepy to talk to him this morning.

"All right, no need to get all huffy," Shade said. Then she pushed her chair back and stood up as if she were leaving. I felt abandoned.

"You're mad?"

She dropped her palms on the table and leaned in close. The musky scent of her skin blended with the freshly ground coffee. It made my ears tingle. "Look, I'm happy you might have work, did you think I wouldn't be?"

Feeling like a big liar, I couldn't answer. I turned my head away as she continued to speak.

"It's not the work, it's that you don't trust me, and, I don't know, the way you act sometimes...what's going on?"

"Nothing's going on," I said, averting my eyes. My lower lip shook, and I was afraid if I said anything I might start crying. Now, I rarely cry and when I do it's not in front of anyone. That would be manipulative.

I glanced around to see if anyone was staring at us, but the people in this casually hip Saturday afternoon crowd were too wrapped up in themselves to notice the force field between Shade and me. Turning my eyes back to Shade, I felt the throbbing in my gums where Dr. Janis had drilled and filled me almost twenty-four hours earlier. The delayed reaction made me feel quizzical, whimsical. I was gushing.

Catching me, Shade's lips softened into a crescent. "Dammit, Slivowitz, what am I going to do with you?"

"I don't know, take me to the movies or something."

"No," she said. "You're the one who got laid last night, you can take me to the movies."

She walked off to the bathroom and left me sitting at the table with my cheeks and ear lobes radiating as if I'd been drinking red wine all morning. My responses to her were becoming so physical, the opposite of last night with Ethan.

I wondered if Shade believed I'd slept with him for work. I could have; I'd slept with men for a lot more. And for less. Sitting here in this noisy café, with the rain coming down and Shade only a few feet away, my reluctance to call Ethan now seemed foolish, counterproductive. A job was a job.

I picked up Shade's cell and called. He answered on the first ring. "Are we okay?" he asked, sounding somewhat brusque.

"Yes," I said.

"You sure?"

"Yes."

"Okay," he said. Then came a few awkward seconds.

"So what's up?" I said.

"Up? What do you mean, up?"

"You said you had work?"

"Oh yeah. Ever hear of Alexis Calyx?"

When I said no, Ethan assured me she was all the rage in some circles, particularly in the oxymoronic adult film industry where she'd won numerous Skin Awards and had become one of the first video-box girls. Apparently, she started her own production company, which produced what she called feminist erotica, material that found her enmeshed in the censorship wars. "She testified at the Meese Commission," he said as if it meant something to him.

"Wait a second, you want a piece on a porn star?"

"No, even better, she needs a ghostwriter. See, she's got this contract for an autobiography and doesn't have time to write, or maybe she's illiterate, who knows? I just met her a couple of weeks ago."

"But I don't know anything about pornography."

"I figured as much," he snickered, and I remembered how much pleasure it had given me when Freddy bit him last night. "Alexis is keen on that, actually. The last ghostwriter turned out to be some sycophantic fan. Freaked the shit out of her."

"This is what I get for sleeping with you," I said. Two women at the next table looked over.

"Here's a novel concept," Ethan said. "Someone does you a favor and you say thank you. Want to give it a shot?"

I was getting ornery with everyone today, wasn't I? I apologized to Ethan and asked for the information. My black roller ball bled into the front page of *The Free Spirit,* upon which I scrawled the name Alexis Calyx and beneath it, her phone number. When I clicked off the phone, I noticed that I'd drawn a few five-point stars around her name. I would soon learn how apt my etchings had been, but for now I repeated the name out loud: "Alexis Calyx." What a brush of palate-licking that wrought, a name spoken in tongues and multiple entendres. I pictured a woman in white taffeta running through fields of blazing grass and dewy, wet flowers. I was going to hate her.

Stepping out of the bathroom, Shade jolted me from Merchant-Ivory dreamland back to the thunderstorms along Ninth Avenue. I tore the name and number from the newspaper and shoved it into my back pocket. With it went all thoughts of porn stars and ex-boyfriends and everyone else around us. My focus was entirely on Shade walking toward me in her velvet hip-huggers as if she were working a runway, smiling as if she knew exactly what I was thinking.

An espresso machine slurped and steamed. Spoons clinked into ceramic cups as couples practiced synchronized stirring. Shade and I were no different. Sitting across from each other again, not saying a word, she drew circles with her finger on the steamy window pane, and together we looked out into the rain, its reverberant pounding a reminder that we were part of something else, just as a lover, even a bad one, can affirm that you still belong to your body.

I turned back to her, saw her floating in a glowing nimbus like the paint-by-number pictures of Christ they sold on the street, and at that second felt as if months...no a lifetime goddammit! I felt as if a lifetime of Novocain was beginning to wear off.

Still Life With Videotape

The Master of Self-Deliverance spoke about his thirty-minute *Docudeath* tape of the Ida and Marvin Salinger suicides. I sat silently, preferring to listen to Kaminsky a while before saying anything myself. I hated being back in this office with its obese metal desks and finger-printed walls, the fiendish glow of the fluorescents, the antiphonal chime of the fax machine. And I was here sans working papers. Last time I'd come as a reporter, when Kaminsky still needed the coverage. I'd felt protected, bivouacked by the same credentials that allowed me entry into worlds I would not otherwise see: Congressional assemblies, a Senator's motel room, towns devastated by natural disasters, crack houses, fairness-in-media conventions, and, most recently, the New York City courthouses. Armed with the First Amendment, the public's right to know, and occasionally a press pass, I could go anywhere, say anything to anybody, and never take no for an answer. On my own, I was too shy to walk into a bar or go to the movies by myself.

"We've just completed the home video copy," Kaminsky said, sitting perpendicular to me in a chair of peeling chrome and yellow-green vinyl. Apparently, orders for the tape were coming in faster than calls to the Home Shopping Network on a bottom price item. He had set up an 800 number and had an intern monitoring the phones. Then there were the television and radio call-ins, the satellite conferences, round tables on the Internet. His was a conundrum fit for the modern MacLuhanite: so many tools, so little time.

All of this and the Attorney General couldn't substantiate any of the charges against him. It didn't hurt that he'd hired a celebrated attorney and an upscale public relations firm, which had leaked snippets of the Ida and Marvin tape. What TV station could resist these cherubic faces telling America that suicide was a lifestyle choice? Hours later came the faxed release stating that proceeds from the video sales would go to medical research foundations.

I couldn't stop thinking of Shade's perfect comment about the suicides being a septuagenarian snuff film. Fidgeting in my chair, I uncrossed my legs, then quickly crossed them the other way. My stomach gurgled in stereo, so I had to speak. "When they came to you..." I said and almost didn't recognize my own voice, "did they know what they wanted?"

"Oh, yes, they knew," he nodded. "You have to, otherwise I won't get involved. There's too much risk."

"You mean legally?"

"At the very least." He stared at me so I looked away. I saw he had hung my jacket from a coat rack frond; a mound of leather protruded in between its shoulders like a Hollywood gun hidden in a suit pocket. That was so bad for the leather.

"You see, Rachel." Hearing my name brought me back, a bit horrified that I returned to him. I had to fight the desire to grab my jacket and run. "You don't mind me using your first name, do you?"

"No, that's okay."

"I simply cannot afford to be wrong. Do you realize how many requests I get a day? And since the suicides, this popularity, I can't tell you...I talk to everyone. You cannot even imagine."

"I'm afraid I can."

"So, we're talking about cancer here?"

I nodded yes, but was tempted to say no. Even sitting in this office with the Master of Self-Deliverance, I had trouble admitting to myself just why I'd come. I thought of Aunt Lorraine at home in bed and wished I was there with her, watching games shows, playing backgammon, keeping this damn disease away from her.

Kaminsky smiled and his deeply creviced face went from dour to distortedly happy. His upper lip twitched. "Cancer is my soft spot. I was once an oncologist, you see? So much pain."

"The thing is I think it's more that she's afraid of dying, than actually...she doesn't want to, to..." I was stalled by a lump in my throat, then surprised at how the words had begun to come out. If I continued to speak, however, I was afraid of what might come next. Where I used to tether my emotions with a performer's professional grace, I felt as if, recently, the reigns had been cut loose.

"I had a patient last year, a lovely woman," Kaminsky said. "She had bone marrow cancer. The way her family talked you would have thought she couldn't make it another day. I met with her a couple of times, we talked. She ended up living almost a full year after that. She took a trip to Belize. Went to her grandson's high school graduation."

I didn't say anything. Just ground my teeth against the rim of the paper cup.

"The reality is, sometimes just knowing I'm here, whether we go through with it or not...it's enough. They say knowledge is power; well in these cases the knowledge that there's help is a measure of control."

"Control? What kind of control can she have on television? I don't want her on television," I blurted out.

"It is quite troublesome."

"But you said you film everyone."

"No, *I* don't film anyone. I simply suggest that people document the process themselves, for their own protection. These are legal questions, not moral. For me the only morality is seeing that each patient gets the death he or she wants. Within that framework if one wishes to take a stand—go on television for instance—so much the better. But it doesn't often happen that way, the logistics alone take months, and, sadly, the segment of the population I'm dealing with doesn't usually have that kind of time."

I stared at him, this little man with his gaunt cheeks and white-gray hair with whom Aunt Lorraine felt kindred because his parents, like her father, had perished in Nazi-occupied Poland. They were survivors long before the word was usurped by talk-show shrinks and twelve-step programs.

"She wants to see you." My eyes welled and my head grew heavier. Looking up, I saw my leather jacket still stretching from frond contact. Noticing it seemed stupid, insignificant, of a different world than Kaminsky and me. I turned back to him, and although I'd expected the twisted glint of a mad scientist, he actually looked sad. As if his face had absorbed my aura.

"I will see her then," he said, and I felt soothed momentarily in his presence. A comfort akin to getting your period after a two-week pregnancy scare, but comfort nonetheless. These days I took whatever I could get.

I breathed deeply, swallowed back a tear as Kaminsky and I matched our filofaxes for a date. Before leaving, I asked if I could buy a copy of the *Docudeath* tape. He handed me a video in a plain white jacket. "Take it," he said. "It's a little bit longer than the ones we're selling."

"The director's cut?"

"Rachel," he put a hand on my shoulder, and I felt a rumbling inside my chest. "You have more strength than you're aware of, you'll see."

I couldn't hold back the tears this time. Kaminsky sat me down again, took my hand. "It's okay, this is all very normal."

"I'm sorry," I hiccuped.

"No apologies." He handed me a tissue, and I blew. Already, I feared needing him too much. I wanted to thank him for his kindness, then tell him I'd made a mistake and would never see him again. But I could only cry incessant streams of tears until the little buggers robbed every ounce of fluid from my body. Through it all, Kaminsky stayed calm.

Outside, I wiped a few crispy leaves from the window of my jeep. Last week's heat wave was a vague memory, repressed by chilly winds and dipping thermometers. Fall in New York had officially begun.

I climbed inside, turned the rear-view mirror toward me. Using a tissue I found on the dashboard, I scraped the lines of mascara from my face. I didn't look that bad. My eyes and cheekbones and mouth all appeared softer than they had in weeks. But I didn't trust my reflection. I blanketed my cheeks and nose with a fresh layer of beige cover-up, and reapplied slightly gothic proportions of black mascara. The engine grumbled to a start, and I was off to meet Alexis Calyx.

At first, the voice on her answering machine had unnerved me. It was so strong and passionate, like a Patti Smith song. Nothing 900-number about it. I hung up twice before finally mustering the courage to leave a message. She picked up as I was talking, which meant she knew it was me who'd hung up before, and therefore had probably surmised I was nervous or a person of strange telephone habits. Not a good start. Now, having just spent an hour discussing Aunt Lorraine's death-bed wish, I was even more unsettled about meeting the porn star. From death to sex in less than thirty minutes. I suppose I was luckier than those who'd gone the other way, people who died accidentally from auto-erotic asphyxiation. Nelson Rockefeller.

I downshifted into the lunchtime gridlock that was Broadway, thinking: what am I doing? Writing a porn star's life was no job for a journalist. Aunt Lorraine would be horrified, and she was the one who'd introduced me to the profession. We used to sit in the basement—before Neil coopted the space as his metal workshop/dungeon—and watch old newsreels on Dad's rickety 8-mm projector. A buddy in the electrician's union had given Dad the newsreels. I loved the beginning shots, with newspapers flying from the presses faster than anything I'd ever seen. Then came the zooming headlines, mostly about World War II and the Holocaust.

As I watched Hitler's face, streaked by the old film, I would ask Aunt Lorraine to tell me the story of her escape.

"Again, you want the story?"

"Please." I batted my eyes, knowing she couldn't resist.

My paternal grandparents had lived in Lodz where my grandfather was a writer, a newspaper man. Early on, he sensed trouble and put his sister, his wife, and her two children on a boat for Argentina, where his own mother had been living for almost ten years. "I remember throwing up a lot," Aunt Lorraine said. "The four of us clung together on that boat with only one blanket for weeks. We ate stale bread until it ran out. Then your father one day came back with a pickle and cut it into four pieces with his pocketknife. I never tasted a pickle so good. At night we slept crowded next to each other and your father, you know his bladder troubles. I worried nobody would let us in the way we stunk."

As she spoke, I saw it all in grainy newsreel images: the ramshackle ocean liner, the itchy wool blanket, my father, Aunt Lorraine, even my grandfather who was shot dead in a Polish ghetto after refusing to stop publishing his newspaper. My family history unraveled in a soundtrack of Polish, Yiddish, and Spanish. Those Sonnanovicz-turned-Slivowitzes with their bizarre migratory patterns had traversed ghettos from Lodz to Buenos Aires, and, finally, ended up in Bay Ridge, a hodgepodge of language, culture, and custom. By the time I was born, nobody knew what came from where. We ate kasha with pinto beans, brisket with Ragu spaghetti sauce. By day I saluted the American flag and sang "God Bless America;" but by night came the mournful sounds of Agustin Magaldi singing "Adios Muchachos" from Dad's lopsided record player.

I remember my father spoke mainly Spanish, preferring its romantic lulls and rolls to the colder, more guttural phonetics of the *shtetls* and to the slippery slang of Brooklyn English. It also came in handy whenever he and Aunt Lorraine didn't want the rest of us to know what they were saying, though this peeved Mom. Not only did she feel excluded, but she herself had come from a long line of German Jews, the Most Favored Nation among the diaspora. Growing up, Mom's voice shadowed me: *You listen, Rachel! We might live with these Slavs, but you must understand the family you come from...you know who they mean when they talk about the chosen.*

Yet, those chosen among the chosen couldn't forgive one of their own for marrying a Polack, and a Polack who moved comfortably through Brooklyn's bodega culture was downright scandalous. Mom lost her MFN status the day she became a Slivowitz. *Marrying for love was my biggest mistake. I was once a Durkheim, and now what? A nasty liqueur...where did they ever come up with that name?*

Later, having my own problems with that name, I would molt the Slivowitz skin myself. But as a young child, before I internalized the undercurrent of self-hatred that follows survival and started passing as Italian, I loved those zany Polacks; my grandmother and great Aunt Ida who fed me sweet babka and smiled, "good girl, good girl;" the brood of chubby-cheeked, hyperactive cousins, all boys, who fought with Rowdy and Neil, although Neil always ended up bruising this cousin's wrist or sending that one home with a bloody nose.

"A shame we Slivowitzes don't make too many girls," Aunt Lorraine used to say. "You're the only one, the only girl. You'll make us proud." I remember her crying the day I received the scholarship to journalism school. It was the only time I ever saw her cry—not even recently, through all of the doctors and chemo, did she shed a tear in front of me—and I knew she thought I was honoring the memory of my grandfather, the newspaper man of Lodz. Although this was partially true, the means by which I secured my Columbia scholarship were questionable enough to weigh heavily on the mind of this "good girl," who needed Aunt Lorraine's approval. I wanted her to be proud of me so I kept quiet about the loose ends.

After a few circles around the neighborhood, I landed an unmetered spot a block away from the East Village address Alexis Calyx had given me. A deep breath. The click of my keys in the door. I hiked my bag over my shoulder and walked beside a row of brownstones in the nip of the afternoon, wondering about Alexis Calyx. What if her office were a sexual heroin den, like something out of *Caligula,* where upon entering she made you remove your clothes as casually as you had to relinquish your shoes in those Japanese restaurants I always avoided? If I wanted to eat with my shoes off, I would stay home. Neither were my clothes coming off. But what if she were the dominatrix type? If she locked me in a pair of handcuffs? Or taunted me with a rattan cane in a game of Singapore sling? I might be forced into something dangerous, like taking the job.

I thought about climbing back into my jeep and going home, although I knew I couldn't. Ethan would kill me, and though I had fantasized about killing him since our unenchanted evening, I couldn't afford him thinking me irresponsible. Pragmatism in personal relationships was a key to success. I believed strongly in not breaking badly, in keeping all files active; you never knew where you might end up, whom you might need.

Case in point: I was walking down the cracked, concrete stairs into the basement storefront that was home to Zipless Pictures. I pressed the doorbell, and it bounded back with a loud ring like the sound from an old rotary phone. Someone buzzed me inside.

She spoke my name, and I recognized her voice, although the woman coming toward me with her hand extended was hardly the sexual commando I'd imagined. Alexis Calyx had thick, dark hair like mine, but pulled to the side with a fashionable clip, and a sweet, omniscient smile which, oddly, made me think of Aunt Lorraine. She wore a black, tailored suit with no shirt underneath and formidable platform boots that gave her about a foot on me. Her skin was a few pigments darker than mine, leading me to believe her roots were Mediterranean, and her body...for the first time in my life I was tempted to say *built like a brick shithouse,* although I had no idea what a brick shithouse was, let alone what one might look like.

Poised, as if my heart were not pounding like a cement drill, I exchanged formalities with her, and followed her past the cluttered desks and shelves stocked with video boxes, around a group of young women, all fully clothed, sitting in front of a TV screen, eating burritos out of aluminum containers and wielding telephones in exasperated importance. They ignored us as we made our way through the railroad flat, passing colorful, geometric spray-paintings, framed movie posters, a few closed doors, and ended up in a small office.

"I'm sorry, I'm a little frazzled," Alexis Calyx said. She sat down behind a functional, Plexiglas desk and sighed. I took one of the leopard-skin chairs on the other side. "I just came from the set. It's a total zoo, my A.D. had a fight with my male lead and bolted. Okay, so Blink can be a prima donna, but this is news? Now I've got to find her, like I'm the goddamn missing persons bureau. If you want something done do it yourself, I know, I know...anyway, it's just one of those days. Coffee?"

"No thanks."

"Good because that machine drives me nuts, you fill it to five, and it gives you two and it tastes like a burnt bagel, I don't know. We don't want coffee, right? What am I going on here for?"

I couldn't help smiling. So, Alexis Calyx was a little neurotic. This talking at warp speed, and like everyone in my family, she followed her words with emphatic hand movements and pushed the envelope on facial expressions. I felt immediately comfortable with her.

"Right," she pointed her index finger at me and looked down. I watched curiously as she moved her iridescent blue fingernails over the shiny white pages in front of her, which I assumed included the resume and clips I'd faxed her. Her lips cracked into a shrewd smile. "So, Brooklyn College?" she said.

"Yeah, I almost went away, but things happened."

"Tell me about it." She put down the resume and looked at me. "I did a semester at Queens, back when I was getting into the business, but, believe me, school was the last thing on my mind. Took me twenty years to get my degree. You grew up in Brooklyn then?"

"I did."

"What part?"

"Bay Ridge."

"Me, I'm just a little Italian girl from Bensonhurst myself, but nothing like Miss Norma Jean or the other one. Shit, who was the other one? Come on, help me out here, *Gentlemen Prefer Blondes?*"

"Jane Russell."

"The Cross Your Heart bra lady, I'm impressed. But I'm hardly from the wrong side of the tracks. So don't you get any ideas." She smiled, and I thought, that's it—Alexis Calyx was the Jane Russell of Bensonhurst, a grown-up version of my youthful wanna-be fantasies. I couldn't help wondering how this little girl from Bensonhurst made it to the front lines of the sex industry.

"I didn't know Brooklyn had any right sides," I tested.

"*Au contraire,* my dear journalist. Sorry to say I had a happy childhood."

"Really? What was that like?"

She laughed. "In due time, all in due time. Today, I get to ask the questions."

I leaned my right elbow back on the chair and said: "Fire away."

She took out a pen and yellow legal pad, then launched into a rapid succession of questions. Whenever I spoke she scribbled on the pad. She asked me who my favorite actor was. I couldn't think of any. Actress? Too tempted to say Jane Russell, I begged off that one as well. Who would I be voting for in the Mayoral election? I never voted, in journalism school some professors said it wasn't entirely ethical. Did I believe politicians had any business messing with people's sex lives? Absolutely not. Interfering with the arts? No way. Regulating pornography? Well...um...maybe when it came to children. Did I have a favorite X-rated film? Aside from fragments on cable television and the original *Last Tango in Paris,* which I hated, I'd never actually seen an X-rated film.

I enjoyed the question-and-answer game and the congenial badinage that stemmed from her queries. It was the easiest job interview ever, and I had to admit she was intriguing, this brick shithouse from Bensonhurst. A bit frazzled, yes, but she was smart in an actions-speak-louder-than-words way, frankly the kind of intelligence I always admired.

"Okay, let's cut to the chase." She put down her pen, locked her fingers beneath her chin, and looked me straight in the eye. "You'd have to watch my erotica, some of the hard core, too. You're okay with that?"

"Sure."

"And come to the set, of course."

"No...I mean, it's no problem." Even if it were a problem, I wouldn't have said anything. I don't know what kind of brain-washing or subliminal seduction was going on in that office, but my do-the-right-thing claims to truth and public service were dwarfed in the presence of Alexis Calyx. I wanted the job with her.

"Brilliant," she beamed, and I wasn't sure whether she meant me or my porno naïveté. Either way, it didn't matter. Nor was I concerned that we spoke no specifics about the job itself. I figured I was in when she started picking through the shelves lined with videotapes, some still masked in plastic, others in generic, white boxes with titles scrawled in black magic marker. She stood on a chair to reach the higher shelves and handed tapes down to me in an assembly line process, during which someone knocked at the door.

"Come in, come in," Alexis said. A red-headed woman in a tight black body suit and jeans inched open the door. We both stared at her. "Well, what is it?"

"Um...Alexis?"

"Yes?"

"You...um, better come here a sec," the young woman said, and they exchanged the kind of tell-all glance that informed me they'd known each other for a while. Alexis jumped down from her chair and turned to me.

"Would you excuse me one moment, please?"

I nodded, "Sure."

I sat down again, glanced around the office. Aside from the rows of tapes kept in their black metal cage behind the desk, the decor was minimalist. A poster for a movie called *Sensurround,* starring the one and only Alexis Calyx, hung by the door. An abstract painting in black, white, and gray covered most of the wall perpendicular to the desk. Opposite the painting were two windows, Levelors pulled up, unveiling a courtyard view of amputated branches, split fences, the backsides of weathered brick buildings with scaly molding, rusted bars covering the lower floor windows, and a few air conditioners bulging like cysts.

Alexis still gone, I turned my attention to the pile of videotapes and thumbed through a few titles: *All the President's Women, It's a Gang-Bang New Year, Sheila and Her Purple Penis, Brothers Do It Deeper.*

I felt as if I'd been yanked from the glamour and excitement of a movie set and deposited in the back alley of Zipless Pictures. I couldn't help but think of my brothers: Rowdy and his random fits of cursing, spitting in my face, or shoving me around; and Neil, who never hit me, but was always drilling holes in my wall or breaking through the dead bolts I put on my bedroom door with a crowbar. Sometimes he showed up under my bed. Other times he left me dead water bugs and pictures of naked girls with an arm or a leg missing. Once, he locked me in a pair of handcuffs and Dad had to cut them off with a huge metal clip.

Neil seemed, like the wounded vets home from Vietnam, lost in maze of contemplative terror that as time went on made him violent and angry; Rowdy, on the other hand, maintained the demeanor of a pathetic, petty criminal. Before going to jail for the first time when he was nineteen, he let me in on one of his schemes. He had tape recorded the sounds that different coins made when they were dropped into a public telephone (*b-b-b-b-buuup* was a quarter, *be-beep* a dime, *boop* a nickel), and dubbed them onto myriad cassette tapes. The system worked like this: You dialed a number, the operator said please deposit X amount for X number of minutes, you put the mouthpiece to the tape deck and pressed play. The sounds registered as real coins.

He rigged it for me one day. We got the number of a hotel in London from the travel section of the paper and dialed. "See, no coins," Rowdy whispered, as he held the receiver to his boom box. Right away, a woman with a thick English accent said, "Hullo!" I made a reservation.

When Neil got wind of Rowdy's Rube Goldberg contraption, he saw greenbacks glowing behind the empty eyes of his older brother. He sent Rowdy peddling tapes through Brooklyn's immigrant communities, while he stayed home counting and dispensing their earnings. Years dealing nickel bags of skunk weed had given Neil the ability to turn a profit on such low-level commodities. At least he was selling the pot himself and not brokering it through his idiot brother.

For months, the cops combed the borough looking for the notorious Telephone Thief until one day they spotted a man standing in a phone booth for hours with a tape deck the size of a traveling suitcase. They brought him in for questioning and, within hours, the cops were ravaging through Rowdy's room where they discovered cassette tapes replete with thousands of *b-b-b-b-buuups, be-beeps,* and *boops.*

Rowdy was sent to Rikers; I went to confession. I'd seen enough movies to know exactly what to do when I walked into that cold, intimidating booth. "Forgive me Father for I have sinned," I said, and then recounted the story of the telephone fiasco, altering enough facts to protect my fraudulent claims to Catholicism. At ten years old I was already quite the little story teller. I talked. The priest listened. Then he blessed me and sent me on my way.

I went back a few times until he started asking me whether I'd accepted the ways of the Lord Jesus. Now, I had no great love of the Jewish religion, which came to me in a genetics of weakness, assimilation, and death, but never did I think of becoming a full-time Catholic. Besides, I couldn't see that confession actually *did* anything. I wanted change, not absolution. I wanted better brothers.

"That's a bit scary, trust me." I was shaken by Alexis' voice; *Brothers Do It Deeper* fell to the floor. Alexis scooped up the tape and walked back behind her desk. "I was such an ingenue back then, so young and stupid. Then again, we all have our crosses, don't we?"

"Oh, yeah," I nodded, still flustered by streaks of childhood.

"Anyway, I'm sorry, but I have to cut this short. My A.D.'s resurfaced with a list of demands. Apparently, she thinks it's Lebanon or something. She runs off my set and has the balls to come back with demands—like I have time for this. I have an exam at five."

"Oh, okay."

"A mid-term no less."

"I thought you finished your degree?"

"You listen, I like that." She set down the tape and stared across the desk at me as intensely as she'd eyed the woman who interrupted our earlier conversation, and, once again, I experienced the subterranean tug of her personality.

She smiled. "You want all the answers, don't you?"

"Just one for now."

"Fair enough. In the real world, my dear scribbler, I'm in law school. I have a torts exam today."

"Wow." I half-laughed, feeling as dumb as my language and a bit out of my league. Alexis Calyx wasn't supposed to be book smart. Interesting, yes. Worldly, sure. But law school?

"What can I say?" Alexis said. "It took me so long to finish my degree I got used to having school in my life. Of course, it's not really that simple, but you know that. Or you will soon."

She turned around and shuffled through the stack of videotapes on her desk, every so often placing one in a pile for me. I watched her shuffle the porno tapes with her glittering fingernails and tried to imagine those same fingers lugging a briefcase full of legal documents downtown. She would have to use a different shade of polish. No lawyer I knew wore iridescent blue.

"You don't mind if I do the contract myself?" she asked as she led me back outside through her industrious minions.

"Not at all."

"Good. I think we're going to get along just fine, Miss Rachel from Bay Ridge. The thing to remember is this is a business like any other....Hey, hey, Alia." She stopped a woman in big brown sunglasses and a tight satin overcoat who must have been about my age. "Un-uh, not on your life. Once shame on you, twice shame on me." The woman laughed as Alexis turned to me. "Rachel, meet Alia, my stellar A.D., the one with demands. I'm surprised you didn't take hostages."

"That's a good idea. Next time."

"Trust me, honey, there will not be a next time. Are you this much trouble over at that Hollywood finishing school?"

"Hollywood finishing school?" I asked. The three of us walked outside into the crepuscular haziness, a cocktail-hour laziness.

The stellar A.D. smirked, "N.Y.U."

"Back in the seventies we would have laughed if anyone came to us from film school, but what's that Dylan line? Come on, help me out here."

"Dylan Thomas?" said the A.D.

"Dylan Bob."

"*The times they are a'changing,*" I said.

"Precisely," Alexis said. "Anyway, we've got to run."

A short goodbye, and I was left standing in front of Zipless Pictures, my arms stuffed with tapes and the draft of an autobiographical essay Alexis was writing for a snappy feminist journal called *Good Witch.* As I skimmed the piece in the shifting rays of sun, the world of Alexis Calyx spurted into my veins. Curiosity, once piqued, was my favorite high. Some reporters got off on the rush of breaking a hot story, and yes, I had to admit it was trippy knowing that people sitting down to their morning coffee would gawk a *holy shit!* gaze over your words. But I was a process junky, more excited by travel than the final destination. By the time I finished a story I was already tracking down the next; rarely did I read my own work in print. One might say I suffered from fear of little death syndrome.

And what of its cure? Years cavorting with post-Freudians—the Kleinian or Lacanian crowd—at one hundred fifty dollars a forty-five minute hour? I don't think so. I simply went on believing that each story might be the one that stopped me dead in my tracks. Forever waiting for the big O.

A few days later, on a crisp Halloween morning, I drove out to Bay Ridge with the *Docudeath* tape and a brand new television set. It was an early Chanukah gift for Aunt Lorraine, a big, fancy model with a built-in VCR. Over the years, after I'd moved to Miami and started making money, I occasionally bought Aunt Lorraine and Mom expensive gifts to assuage my guilt for leaving. I wasn't about to let the strike break me of this habit, at least not while I still had credit cards and Aunt Lorraine was stuck with a set so old the figures swelled and released as if they were controlled by invisible sound waves. Aunt Lorraine said she didn't mind, that she felt as if she were watching life through a kaleidoscope. That was when she could still make it downstairs for anything important, cop shows or *Press Talk.*

I paid two boys who lived across the street five dollars each to carry the set inside and up to Aunt Lorraine's bedroom. Rowdy followed silently behind, eyeing them nervously as they dragged the set across the rug and over to the foot of Aunt Lorraine's bed.

"Wow!" The smaller boy jumped back upon noticing Aunt Lorraine, who was asleep with a dry, white tongue hanging against her lower lip, and her eyelids twitching. "How'd her face get so puffy?"

"Cancer," I said.

"Oh," he nodded sagely, as if he should have known from her greenish skin tone and the IV tube plugged into her arm. He nudged his brother out of the room, and I realized it was the tube that sent jitters so deep inside my stomach I couldn't eat for hours after I'd been here.

Aunt Lorraine had once been the most vibrant woman I knew: always reading and talking and asking questions long before Alexis

Calyx had even left Bensonhurst. Who was the greatest American president? Franklin Delano Roosevelt. Why did so many Nazis flee to Argentina? Because that's where the Jews were hiding. Until recently, I always knew the answers she wanted to hear.

Apparently, she'd had a feeling about the cancer for some time but kept it to herself. Only when the lump in her breast grew as big as a golf ball did she acquiesce to seeing a doctor, who turned her over to an oncologist. Both of her breasts were removed; she underwent chemotherapy. But it was too late. About a month ago, they found that the cancer had infiltrated her bones.

Mom said Aunt Lorraine's bedroom was starting to smell like a nursing home, a peculiar statement coming from a woman who never stepped foot inside of a nursing home. When her own mother lay dying at Sunset Estates, and I sent her plane tickets to come to Miami, each time Mom succumbed to one of her fainting spells and was unable to visit. Death, Mom said. She knew its scent and it made her nervous. It also gave her cause to tap a mother lode of antidepressants and spa in New Jersey with her gentleman friend, Hyman Hogan. Thankfully, Rowdy was around to clean Aunt Lorraine's commode and change her IV unit or bandages when the nurse wasn't there.

Looking at him sitting on the edge of Aunt Lorraine's bed with his clammy face and those big yellow stains under the arms of his T-shirt, I thought it odd that at the age of forty my balding, dim-witted brother had become Florence Nightingale.

He caught me staring at him. "How'd you know about Beta site anyway?"

"The what?" I squinted as if focusing on him might give me some insight into his world.

"See it's got the test scanner on it." He walked over to me and pointed to the panel of buttons on the television set. "You know like in the supermarket how they got those scanners, right? Well, a lot of people don't know this, but they can read your brain with them, but only if you got implants. They started with dogs, and then they moved on to people, prisoners first. That's where I got mine. In prison."

"Do I have one?"

"Nah, only people who been down by the government," he said. He walked back to the bed and sat down, bugging his eyes back and forth between Aunt Lorraine and me. "It's going to blow up when she sleeps," he said.

"Don't worry, I know how to hook up a TV." Despite the various instruction manuals and stray wires all over the floor, I knew what I was doing. It was an ego thing that I had a handle on technology. My father was the autodidactic electrician, after all.

Rowdy laughed hysterically, his mouth open so wide I could see all of his missing teeth. "No, I mean Aunt Lorraine." He held both of his hands over his stomach. "Her face blows up when she sleeps." I had to laugh along with him. "Then, she starts shrinking and by the end of the day she's a skeleton like the faces they got in the drug store, you know, for Halloween. Oh man, she's so sick..." his voice tapered off, and I watched a tear drip from the corner of his eye.

"It's okay," I said.

"No way, man. You don't know." His voice was getting contentious.

"Please. Let's not fight about it."

"I'm the one who takes care of her," he cried. "You don't know nothing!"

"What's it she don't know that you think you know?" Mom said. I had no idea how long she'd been standing in the doorway watching me hook up the television set.

"Hello, Mom," I said.

She smiled slyly beneath her creamy brown bouffant and walked toward me, turning her cheek for me to kiss it. She smelled sickly sweet, like Poison or Opium. "And what's this?" she said.

"It's a television."

Rowdy was flustered. "Both of you don't know dogshit, I'm the one who's here all the time."

Mom ignored him. She'd been jealous of Rowdy since he became a credentialed schizophrenic, robbing her of the family's Most Mentally Ill title. I thought she had it all wrong; his illness, if anything, gave credence to her own.

"I know *what* it is," Mom said. "How did it get here?"

"I bought it for Aunt Lorraine."

"Rachel's some big spender now. No job, but she's buying TVs and you, what do you care? You're off in Atlantic City—"

"Shut up, Rowdy."

"Atlantic City?" I said. "I thought you hated gambling."

"We're not talking about me."

"They go for that Merv Griffin stuff. You know, Ma likes the shows."

"Look, there's nothing wrong with me spending some time with my boyfriend."

"Boyfriend," I said. "You're almost sixty-five years old, you don't have a boyfriend."

"Maybe she's jealous," Rowdy said. I ignored him this time.

"Look, don't you blame me that you can't keep a man," Mom said. "I'm sick of all your projecting."

"What do mean, projecting? I don't project!"

Just then, Aunt Lorraine's eyes opened. I jumped up onto the bed with her and took her hand. Though frail and bony, it felt like one of Ethan's suits, cut from the most expensive silk. "How's the patient?"

"Lousy. They've got me on more pills than...look at them..." she motioned to a tray of plastic containers on the side table, "red, yellow, blue, I'll tell you something. I stopped taking them."

"She thinks she's her own doctor already," Rowdy said.

"You really should take your pills."

"I'm sick of being a Jell-O head," she said, then looked over my shoulder. "What the heck is that thing?"

"She says it's a television set," Mom said.

"I can see, but why? I liked my old TV."

I let go of her hand and huffed. "Forget it, I'm leaving—"

"No no, honey, I love it." Aunt Lorraine winked at me, eyes glistening like the old days. "Come, come, did you bring my tape?"

I nodded, standing up to get the tape out of my bag.

"What's it she's got there?" Mom asked.

"Oh, you know, it's the death video I wanted to see," Aunt Lorraine said.

"The what!" Mom arched her eyebrows, Gloria Swanson-like as usual.

"The one from the television program—Rachel knows that Doctor Kaminsky."

"She knows him," Mom said. "You know him, that monster?"

"I was covering him, I told you that."

"You did not!" Mom said. "And why do we have to watch it, I don't know which one of you is crazier than the other. Have some respect for the dead, would you?"

Aunt Lorraine shrugged. The *Docudeath* video burned against my fingertips. I'd already seen it once, and though it was tastefully done in a tear-jerking, save-the-children sort of way, there was no doubt that it was a step-by-step guide to suicide.

First, however, we experimented with the television set. I showed Aunt Lorraine how to flip the channels, program the split screen, set the clock and timer. No flashing 12:00 in this bedroom. Excited as Aunt Lorraine was, it was the video she'd been waiting for.

I dropped the tape in the VCR and looked at Mom. "Are you all right?"

She shrugged this time.

"Look, Stella," Aunt Lorraine said. "If you don't want to watch, go downstairs."

"Leave now or forever hold your peace," Rowdy said.

"I don't like it at all," Mom said. She pulled up the chair next to Aunt Lorraine's bed and sat down.

Aunt Lorraine, clinging to the remote, pressed play, but instead of Ida and Marvin, what appeared on the twenty-five-inch, precision-image screen was a couple of women, one lying naked on a wet, ceramic tile floor, the other, dressed in a French maid's uniform, caressing with red fingernails the passive woman's stomach, moving up, and up, and up, following slowly with her mouth until she came to the woman's nipples, hard as finely cut diamonds, and her tongue wended its way between them, in long, lulling licks that caused the supine woman to scream out above the stringy soundtrack. Off to the side, a tan, mustachioed man sporting button-fly bell-bottoms and a bad haircut watched intently, his dark eyes conveying a sense of longing so real I found myself identifying with him.

"Ida and Marvin must have had some life," Aunt Lorraine said. Her attention was fixed to the screen.

I jumped up to stop the tape.

"Is this your idea of a joke?" Mom said.

"No, it's not a joke." I turned to face her. "And don't look at me like I'm some kind of pervert. It's research, for a job. I brought the wrong tape."

"Matter of opinion," Aunt Lorraine said. I frantically searched the top of the TV set for the off button. Couldn't find it.

"What do you mean, work?" Mom said. "What kind of work are you doing?"

"Stop the tape! Where's the damn remote?"

"She got it," Rowdy pointed to Aunt Lorraine. He smiled, "Man-O-Manischevitz, Rachel, I never knew you were so cool."

I rolled my eyes. "You can shut it off, Aunt Lorraine...Aunt Lorraine?"

No use. She was hooked. I continued to search for another off button.

"Man, this is classic," Rowdy murmured. "Must be at least twenty years old."

"How do you know that?" I asked him.

"Shit, everyone knows *Sensurround.*"

I took a few steps backward. So this was the infamous *Sensurround,* starring Alexis Calyx and Robbie Rod, her ex-husband, who had also directed the film. It was a parody of those seventies disasters like *Earthquake* and *The Towering Inferno.* I remembered the poster Alexis had hanging on her wall. Then, a fragment from her effusive, confessional essay: "*the sexual choreography runs so close to the apocalypse.*"

With the world crashing to its grand finale, desire reigned supreme. Everything was sex. Raw sex. Desperate sex. Slippery, condomless, big-death/little-death sex. The kind of sex I'd never had. The kind of sex I craved.

On screen, the French maid kissed the naked woman, whom I now recognized to be Alexis. A storm thunderbolted outside the window next to them. The man (Robbie Rod) was naked, too. His penis was absurdly large, the biggest I'd ever seen.

A flash of silver lightning smashed through the window, sending shards of glass sparkling through the air. The music grew somber.

Crescendo speeding up with an accent on the horns. The French maid was gone. Alexis and Robbie Rod lay together, his back to the floor and she on top of him. His toes curled against her right knee cap. The gesture seemed too intimate for this kind of movie, for any kind of movie.

But I couldn't stand another minute of it now. Here. With Aunt Lorraine watching studiously, Mom pretending not to, and Rowdy talking back to the screen. It could have been the *Docudeath* or *Shoah* or any Hollywood action film for that matter. I got up to leave.

"Where do you think you're going?" Mom said. "You still haven't told us—"

"That woman, Alexis Calyx, I'm ghostwriting her autobiography."

Mom frowned, disaffectedly. As if I'd somehow disappointed her by not claiming to be at least a consumer of porn if not a porn star myself. "What's the matter, not scandalous enough for you?"

"Jeeze, you hit the big time," Rowdy said.

Mom didn't think so. "Can't you find any nice people to write about?"

"Nice, who's nice?"

"You used to be. We put you in little dresses."

"Get over it, Ma. She ain't your dress-up doll no more."

Our words were stymied by a stereophonic boom rising from the TV speakers. Another window came crashing down on top of Alexis and Robbie Rod. They fucked obliviously, wholeheartedly, apocalyptically. My thoughts came in fragmented clichés. Goodbye cruel world. Out with a bang and not a whimper. For forty days and forty nights. He died with a smile on his face.

Robbie Rod stood, his back a mosaic of blood and broken glass. He took his penis in his hand and it was as if he were grabbing a thick pole. I couldn't believe that thing had been up inside of Alexis without bruising her internal organs. But she showed no outward signs of damage. She looked up at her man, reverently, part damsel in distress, part lady in waiting. I bolted from the room before the final shot. Before the easy come moment had gone.

One in the Hand,
Two in the Bush

"Hold it!" Alexis commanded. A click and the cameras stopped; all eyes turned to her. Bodies stilled off set as if she'd pressed a pause button. On set, a man relaxed his grip on a woman's thighs, which had been posed missionary-style making her look somewhat like a roasted chicken. Her legs dropped to the bed. He took a few steps back, glaring at Alexis as he stroked his erect penis. But for the alacrity of his hand-cock motion, he looked like some kind of sex zombie.

Having arrived just a few minutes earlier, I took the opportunity to move in and claim a camouflaged spot behind a couple of leafy floor plants, going for my usual fly-on-the-wall routine. Alexis sighed, "Billie, you've got to get the light in closer." Without a word, the woman standing behind a massive eyeball of a light dollied forward. I held out my microcassette recorder. "That's it, on top of her, I want to see her pussy glow. And can we get some glitter makeup on her thighs?" A woman with enough unguents to paint the cast of *Cats* came running. As if she were a gynecologist, she sat down in front of the star's legs and began her cosmetic doctoring. "Beautiful," Alexis said. "We're going for broke here, boys and girls, the fucking of the gods." There were a few giggles. Alexis turned to the naked man. "Mark, don't look at the camera so much. Use your tongue for a while, then pull back and pick up the crystal. Okay, heat 'em up and action!"

Mark, tongue jutting lizardlike from his mouth, moved along the woman's thighs. Two video cameras hovered close to their bodies. The woman moaned, giving what seemed like a virtuoso "*oh, baby, oh!*" I tried to remember her name. It began with a T, Tessa something...Tessa Toupee or Tepee or Tempe. And he must be Mark Vladimir, the featured male lead on this latest Zipless Pictures project: *One in the Hand, Two in the Bush.* It was already being hailed by the Alexis acolytes as groundbreaking erotic cinema.

I took my reporter's notebook from the pocket of my blazer, slipped the ball-point pen from behind my ear, and wrote down a few fragments: Cameras. Smoke machine. Attractive young people with props; clipboards, cell phones, beepers, headphones. Everyone watching. Me watching them watch. The sanctioned voyeur.

Indeed it was like watching the trials I'd covered before the strike, and just as I'd been conscious of researching every case to the last detail I'd come prepared for my virgin viewing of this sex shoot. I'd seen a few videos, skimmed through insider magazines with names like *Skin, Video X-tra,* and *The Bondage & Discipline Tour.* I read selections from the classic texts, everything from Freud and Krafft-Ebing to *The Filmmaker's Guide to Pornography.* Going on-line, I logged into the appropriate newsgroups, gleaning information on new releases, industry feuds, HIV rumors, while familiarizing myself with the jargon. I could tell you the difference between meat and money shots, tout the industry's preference for Astroglide over other lubricants, and delineate scenes by their reductive categories: the boy-girl, the girl-girl, the boy-girl-girl, and so forth and so on.

The category of the moment was boy-girl, the action, post-insertion with sex toy, as Mark moved a thick, conelike crystal in and out of Tessa's vagina, stopping every few minutes to roll his tongue along the clear, wet stick. As they spoke I jotted down their dialogue.

Tessa says: Move me, fuck me with the light of God.
Mark says: Baby, I'm here. I am God.
Tessa says: Oh, I want you inside me now!

Mark took a step back and ripped open a condom wrapper. It was a Zipless rule that couples practice safe sex, HIV test or not, yet there were exceptions: the married couple, the long-term lovers, or women with women who outright refused to work with those silly dental dams. But Mark and Tessa were a nonexception couple. That even I noticed this couldn't be good. No wonder Alexis looked dyspeptic, as if she were on the verge of bursting into bitter song; if this were indeed a musical and not a sex film shoot. The rest of the crew seemed constipated, watching nervously as Mark, a hirsute figure with a penis about the length and width of the average-size banana, fixed an airhole at the end of his condom, smiling perfunctorily at Tessa, whose face, though done up like a side-show gypsy, conveyed a fuck-me-yes-but-I-don't-have-to-like-it quality. Was it me or did she appear sorrowful beneath her rough and tumble exterior? I couldn't stop staring at the bottoms of her feet. Black from stomping back and forth on the dusty wood, they would need a touch of air brushing in the edit suite. The condom wrapper fell to the floor, sounding a light slap. Then came a collective sigh of relief as Mark, penis erect and snugly encased, put his palms on Tessa's thighs and pushed them upward. One camera clung to their torsos, the other moved to Tessa's face. Mark took his penis in his right hand and guided it inside of her.

"Okay," Alexis said, "pickup with the other camera, keep going, on their faces. Good, good...shit! Tessa, be a goddamn martyr if you have to, but don't look like one. Cut!"

As from the sudden burst of a water balloon, frustration splattered in every direction. "We're going to be here forever," a guy in faded jeans, with headphones and a boom mike mumbled to nobody in particular.

"Shut up," Tessa snapped at him. "He smells like onions. I mean once or twice, but this is too much, and he's all soft again. You try smiling about fucking a slinky."

"You think you smell so great with all that flowery crap you rub on," Mark said. "She wonders why I lose my concentration."

"I thought the onions were supposed to help," Tessa whined, as if she were a Class A tattle-tale. I wondered if she had older brothers.

"What is with the onions?" Alexis asked.

"He says they make him more vee-rile," Tessa sneered at him.

"That's not what I said, you little...uh!" Mark jerked his head back in disgust, ran his right hand through his hair, and then glowered back at Tessa. His Adam's apple bobbed up and down as he started to speak. "I said they make my cum more milky."

Alexis quickly moved between them, taking Mark by the elbow. "Look, we're wrapping today, and I absolutely refuse to be here all night. So go brush your teeth and no more onions. What do you do, eat them raw?"

"Like an apple," he said.

Alexis shook her head. "Honey, next time you're worried about the plumbing try zinc capsules like everyone else. Now, you want to clear the set?"

"That's not the problem."

"Yeah right," someone murmured.

"Okay, enough from the peanut gallery. If you want to help, do a private little rain dance for Mark, and you," Alexis turned to Tessa, "go use your vibrator a few minutes. You're being paid to fuck a slinky if you have to."

Alexis sighed, leaned back in her director's chair. She caught my eye and motioned for me to join her. I did as instructed, like everyone else. For as plagued by perfectionism as Alexis was, when she said cut, no matter how long they'd been shooting, everyone stayed with her vision. I got the feeling they all believed they were doing important work, trekking beyond the traditional porno métier...where no *man* had gone before. Women worked cameras, carried cell phones, and swung mikes. Yet even for these millennial years, it veered toward parody. A vision of Lesbos within the drab fascism of California porn.

And where on the Left Coast would you find a director who treated her actors and crew as if they were her own children? The other day I heard her on the phone asking Mark if he'd taken his Cs—he had a cold coming on; now she was pained by Tessa's phallophobia.

"I just don't get it," she was telling me. "I love using her because she doesn't have implants and her tits aren't that big, it's a different kind of aesthetic. It says something. You're recording this?"

I nodded.

"Don't," she said, rubbing two fingers on each of her temples. "I'm too riled, I have to think it through."

"Why are you so upset?"

"Why? I have a feature star who flips out when a man gets near her and you ask, why? Girl-girl scenes she's the best, but this isn't a lesbian company, that's not all we do. I've been telling her she doesn't have to feature, which would be a shame because every time she's on screen, it breaks ranks. She's not what a porn star should look like, blah, blah, semiotic bullshit maybe...but it's true."

"Because she's flat-chested?"

"Yes, of course. But if she won't do men, it's less powerful. Women don't have the tit fetish, most of them anyway. And that's not the point here. She made such a big deal about not wanting to be pigeonholed, not wanting to be an industry dyke. A lot of women are like that, they'll only do girl-girl scenes. It's safer, they feel less pressured with women."

"Less pressured, that's a laugh," I said.

Alexis looked at me, her brow furrowing inquisitively. "Are you a lesbian?"

"No."

She eyed me suspiciously and within seconds I was ten years old again, running to confession for a crime I didn't commit.

"Really, I'm not," I said.

"I'm sensing something, a sort of karmic sound bite. Are you in therapy?"

"Been out a few years, thank you very much." That question was easily answered. As far as I was concerned I'd fulfilled my quota on shrink time with Sam in Miami.

"Then you must have hit on this?" Alexis said, eyebrows raised as if she were waiting for a salacious disclosure. I became conscious of my tight-fitting blazer, the double-breasted wool jacket that wasn't exactly power suit material, but had been conservative enough to get me through the courts. Here it felt constricting, and heated up the back of my neck as if I were hiking the Stair Master. Besides, all the lights and cameras and action had made the set extremely hot.

Think journalism, I told myself. I am a journalist. My job is asking questions. Ask a question. I squeezed into my reporter's face, the one where my brow caverned in between my eyes and my lips pursed downward. "So what happens if Tessa won't do it?" I ventured.

"Oh, she'll do it, she just needs a little tender loving care. Anyway, forget her for the moment. I want to know what's got you so flustered."

"I'm not flustered."

"You are too. The second I asked if you were a lesbian your entire face changed."

"It did not."

"You should see yourself, your cheeks are all red."

"It's hot in here, aren't you hot?" A bead of sweat dripped down the side of my face.

"Heat is an emotion."

I laughed out loud. "That's ridiculous. Heat is a physical condition."

"Brought on by emotion."

"Or temperature."

"The temperature in and of itself is irrelevant. Unless you're moving through it or self-combusting, you don't feel the heat. This is basic physics. So what's got you all worked up? What's making you feel the heat, so to speak?"

"I don't know, maybe the goddamn klieg lights."

"And why?"

"Because they're hot."

"What if I told you the lights were shut off ten minutes ago?"

"Were they really?"

"Immaterial."

"Of course it's material, you just said what if. I have the right to know whether we're speaking hypothetically or not."

"That is exactly my point. We're not talking about the lights, we're not talking about the heat, we're not talking about any physical characteristic of the set. We are talking about why when I asked if you were a lesbian you got flustered."

"I am not flustered!" I shouted, heat brimming beneath my skin, a mockery of my argument. Whatever argument that was. Confused, and embarrassed by the force of my words, I turned my head the other way. Across the set, a group of young women sat laughing and smoking cigarettes. Their easy communication made me angry. So free and libertine they were, working on a radical porno film. I felt even more isolated, more protective of my own world.

Alexis put her hand on my shoulder. "I didn't mean to upset you. I have too many freaked-out people around here already."

"I'm not freaked out." I turned to face her. "It's just that this ghostwriter thing won't work if you keep asking the questions."

"But it's only fair. Yesterday I talked for three hours about my adolescent masturbation to *Playboy.* All I'm asking for is a little reciprocity."

"The more you know about me, the less you'll trust me. I lose my authority."

"You have no authority, Rachel, you work for me."

I stared at her eyes, the folds around them conferring an air of wisdom earned the hard way. Times like these she looked her forty-two years, distinguishable from the rest of her cast and crew, from me, too. She took her hand from my shoulder and tapped my thigh twice, letting her palm linger a moment on my leg. The gesture wasn't at all sexual; it was, in a word, maternal. "All I'm saying is stop being so rigid, this isn't some dumb news story—no offense. Whatever you lose, who cares? Look at what you might gain." Her voice was a combination of brass and silk, it was a *Penthouse* spread transported to the New York Philharmonic, and it provoked the same mesmerizing power I'd felt upon our first meeting, the baptismal belief that my life would be incomplete were I not her ghostwriter. What I hadn't realized was just how unfulfilled I'd been until then. Something like a ghost.

"I really don't want to talk about me," I said finally.

"Oh, I think you do, you've just never been able to. You haven't felt safe."

"You know, I can get this kind of self-help crap anywhere. I didn't have to come to a porno film."

"Say what you like, but it's true. Do you know how many times I've been called a pervert? And practically anytime anybody reviews one of my films I'm mistaken for a whore, but this is what I do, it's who I am. When you're honest with yourself, it makes no difference what anyone else says."

"Just measure it in inches, right?"

"Pardon me?" She studied me as if I were speaking a different language. I'd forgotten how sensitive this industry could be about measurements.

"That's...uh...Warhol," I said, my ears tingling at the silent valleys in between my words. "He...you know, he said you shouldn't read your own press...just measure it."

"I've been saying that for years and I never even knew him. Some of my friends did back in the seventies, but how did you know that? Did you know him?"

"No!" I almost laughed out loud, imagining Andy Warhol coming to Bay Ridge for Thanksgiving dinner.

Alexis tilted her head back and forth. Watching her, the weight of my own hair grew heavier. I tucked it back behind my ears, one side at a time. "Rachel," she said, "if there's one thing I know—well, of course, I do know more than one thing—but I'm an expert on people." She took a deep breath, and I thought if we were part of the movie she would have taken a drag from a cigarette for effect. Instead she made a quick surveillance of the set. The young women were still laughing, a miasma of shimmering hair and cigarette smoke, the man in jeans fiddled with the knobs of a sound mixer, a woman with a clipboard sipped from a paper cup rimmed with big cherry red lipstick stains.

"You can see how being a student of human nature helps in this business," Alexis said, still scanning the set as if we were sitting together at a basketball game.

"No doubt." I feigned sophistication, but my words reverberated self-consciously.

Alexis pivoted toward me. "What I'm saying is, I've been watching you. You hide behind your one-liners, your facts and pithy insights. Believe me, I know irony feels like a safe space, but it's not. You're entitled to your emotions, Rachel. Especially the heated ones."

I felt a disabling sensation, like gas pains. In just a few minutes, Alexis Calyx had managed to disrupt the entire journalistic relationship. If anything, a reporter was supposed to remain emotionally disconnected. Alexis should know better. She'd been interviewed hundreds of times before, even once by Kim Mathews, the doyenne of TV interviewing and perhaps the country's most recognizable journalist, though I use that term loosely.... I stopped myself, for I was indeed making light as she'd accused me of doing, but also because I realized just how flimsy my credentials were around here. I felt like Tessa Tureen, splayed with my dirty feet in the air.

Any real world concerns had spilled out into the East Village streets, while within the studio's sound-proof walls was a greenhouse of possibility. I could have known Andy Warhol. I could be gay. I could be anything I wanted here.

I clutched the back of my neck, wet with perspiration, and stared at Alexis. Our faces were indeed similar, oval shaped, with dark brown, hard-to-manage hair and black coffee eyes; just two little girls from the biggest of boroughs. We shared the ineffable bond of a Brooklyn childhood, just as Aunt Lorraine and Kaminsky together conjured ghosts of Nazi-occupied Poland. In spite of my anger at her invasiveness, as well as her reckless disregard for the tenets of my profession, I was drawn to her. A sensual telotaxis I could barely contain, let alone control.

"I'm too old for this," I said.

"Please, then I'm a dinosaur." She tapped once more at my thigh, and I wanted to tell her about the time Neil locked me in the handcuffs. How I was more afraid of telling on him, of what he might do next, than I was of the restraint. Before I could say anything, however, Alexis and I were interrupted by Alia the A.D. Everyone was set to go. Alexis stood up and winked at me, "Watch closely, this is the take."

My eyes trailed her as she walked toward Tessa, all dolled-up in her red teddy and g-string combo. Alexis leaned her elbows on the star's shoulders. Their eyes locked, Alexis talking and occasionally slipping a couple of fingers through Tessa's strawberry blond hair. The doe-eyed porn star looked almost innocent, an admirable feat given her attire. Again, I felt the encumbrance of my own clothing. Next time I would wear jeans and a T-shirt like everyone else.

Tessa's bare arms locked around Alexis' crisp, white V-neck. Alexis towered over her, stroking her hair. They could have been mother and daughter. Who else would hug her half-naked child that closely? I thought of my own mother, and how I couldn't remember her once putting her arms around me. All my life I'd been waiting for the repressed memory that would prove me wrong.

I felt slightly put off. A little bit of sibling rivalry. Or perhaps the roots went deeper. For they could have been mistaken as lovers, Alexis and Tessa, their bodies entwined in what seemed a comfortable power imbalance.

Alexis gave Tessa's butt a light tap the way football players do after a huddle and then clapped her hands: "Okay, let's get on with it." Tessa flashed her a final adoring look, and I wondered if she was a lesbian. I remembered reading that lesbianism among women off set was as common as men with plumbing problems on it. Somehow, this made sense.

Yet we were all soon shrouded in the shadows of heterosexuality. Only the white of Mark and Tessa's skin shone in cones of amber light. Even Alexis had stepped back as the scene fell into formation. Mark, his limbs sparkling as if they'd been dipped in a barrel of glitter makeup, had no erection trouble. Tessa, too, was more accommodating, her face a blush of lust and satisfaction, her body in tune with Mark's thrusting. Their rhythm was a modern ballet for an unknown audience.

You could smell it, too; the soured lotion, the sweat, the onions, the sex. It came to me in a craving so ignited, so aching, so incomprehensible, I felt myself blush. And I was pulled toward Tessa, this woman with her body arched and head thrusting back and forth. A clump of hair snagged across her mouth, and Mark without taming their beat moved his fingers to her face and gently pushed it away. His touch was so private, so spontaneous, and the way they eyed each other, as if love might be the byproduct of sex and not the other way around, made me envious. Seeking solace, I looked around the audience as if staking out the faces of fellow movie-goers, trying to gauge...what? If anyone else was moved by this? If anyone was aroused by it? Ashamed of it? Part of me wanted to giggle childishly...*these people are fucking!* Yet another part wanted to jump into the scene, to lick Tessa's nipples, to suck Mark's penis, and sandwich myself between them, the three of us thrashing and burning until we all collapsed in a nest of exhausted arms and legs.

Mark, sweat dripping from his rosy face, shouted, "I'm going to come." Tessa screamed back at the top of her lungs. No words, just a series of loud grunts that had me leaning forward with my eyes shut, slipping into the heat, the motion, a desire so palpable it dripped down my limbs. I could barely catch my breath. Mark screamed, "Oh baby, I'm coming!" I slipped backwards, my eyes shot open. Mark fell on top of Tessa and his breathing slowed...and her breathing slowed...and my breathing slowed....

Alexis, face glimmering proudly, screamed, "Cut!" I leaned against a folding chair, still captivated by the naked bodies on set. So at ease in the aftermath, they gave the impression of being a long-married couple. Next to them I felt almost prepubescent.

Mark jumped up and shook out his hair. "That was so hot," he said, giving Tessa's forehead a light kiss. "Did you want to come?"

"In front of all these people, are you kidding me?" Tessa stood up and purred a round of thank-yous to the crew parting beside her with coos and compliments as she retired to her dressing room. A job well done.

And she didn't come. And nobody found this strange or incomplete. Nobody questioned her womanhood, suggested analysis, or stomped with iron feet back and forth, trying to resolve those issues that would set her orgasm free. She walked off the set even more of a diva for not coming. The next time anyone complained about me not coming I would say I was a porn star.

The idea stayed with me as I waited for Alexis amid the end-of-day collapsing of the set. Before today I would have thought my breasts too small, but they weren't any smaller than Tessa's. Maybe I wasn't as skinny as Tessa, but I wasn't exactly fat. Actually, I was in pretty good shape for a woman just over thirty who hadn't been to the gym in a few weeks. I would work out more. I would also need a few glasses of wine, or—who am I kidding?—I would need a couple of Quaaludes before I could take my clothes off in front of all those people. No wonder most porn stars used pseudonyms.

Perhaps, then, it was someone else people were ogling at, panting with, masturbating over.

Alexis herself had adopted a whole new identity upon entering the industry; few people were aware her real name was Patricia DeFabio. If I were to take a name, I would keep something of myself in it: maybe Rachel Sliver or Rachel Slipper. No, I liked the word silver, its prurient shine, the way it bit back when you had it in between your teeth. And it was all mine, the name I'd chosen myself on my eighteenth birthday. Silver...like the chrome of the klieg lights, the glint from Hi-8 lenses, the beams, the rays, those silver rays...oh, yes, Silver Ray...sweet sobriquet. *One in the Hand, Two in the Bush* staring Mark Vladimir, Tessa Touche, and Silver Ray.

Yes, I could be a porn star if I wanted to.

I whispered the name Silver Ray until Alexis came to fetch me. Though giddy with my new identity, I was silent on the way back to the office where Alexis said she had a few "special" videotapes for me.

"I'm looking for my favorite girl-girl scene," Alexis said, pulling tape after tape from the shelf. Apparently, she thought she knew my sexual secret, although I had neither confirmed nor denied it myself. Oddly enough, I didn't mind. Having lesbian tendencies seemed an asset among this crowd. "It's an important theme for us, subversively that is," she said. "Time to steal it back from the boys and their computer-generated fantasies—it's like they keep remaking the same triple-X version of the Victoria's Secret catalogue. All of those shaved pussies and long red fingernails, please...and then they Vaseline the lenses to make everything so soft and dreamy. Have you ever seen women fuck each other? I mean really fuck each other, it's—" She paused, turning her head over her shoulder as if to make sure she still had my attention. Caught in her stare, I felt the heat of the set return to my cheeks, only this time I was more fed-up than embarrassed. I wanted to tell her I'd had enough, tell her I'd grown weary from her little theories on feminism and film and sexuality and shaved pudenda. I wanted to go home.

Perhaps she sensed my discomfort, or she'd fallen upon her own internal censors, for at that very moment she said she didn't want to prejudice my thinking *before* I watched the film. She swung her head back around and continued with the tapes until she found a box with the title *X-posure* scrawled along the spine.

"Here's my baby." She handed me the tape, along with a few others. I took them in exchange for the four tapes I had in my bag.

"You don't mind if I hold onto *Sensurround?*" I asked. The truth of it was Aunt Lorraine wanted it. She said it made her laugh, brought back memories. Memories? Nobody had those kind of memories, but I couldn't ask her to elaborate.

"Ah, *Sensurround,*" Alexis sighed theatrically. "It's brilliant, isn't it? Robbie's swan song."

"Really?"

"Well, he still acted, but...." She leaned her hand on the doorway and looked up in her thinking-woman's pose. "They say it's dangerous for an artist to know success too early. And that's what he was back then, an artist. He wasn't like the others, never a one-day wonder man. After *Sensurround* they all called him Orson Welles; then they crucified him for it." She turned to me, a faraway gaze in her eyes as if she were vacationing in the seventies. "I fell in love with him because of that movie. Bastard."

"Is he?"

She smiled slyly. "Show me a man with a twelve-inch cock who isn't."

"Jesus, that's bigger than Barbie."

She shut off the light, led me out of her office, and although only a few minutes earlier I'd been eager to leave, the way she spoke of her ex-husband had roused my curiosity. Yet as much as I wanted to keep the conversation going, say something more about measurements perhaps, I experienced the strange sensation of stumbling down a dark street and coming to a well-lit diner, but as I went for the door a hand turned the sign from Open to Closed. Alexis Calyx and I were through for the day.

Before *X-posure,* I'd been looking without touching. But I did get aroused, omnivorously so. There was no telling which scenes might catch my fancy: boy-girl, girl-girl, girl and her large electronic appliance....Pleasuring myself, however, seemed disrespectful to Alexis. She was my employer, her videos part of my research.

Yet, by handing me a film she believed was tailored to my specific desire, Alexis Calyx had in fact given me permission to indulge myself. Twisted logic, indeed; perhaps the residue of my two or three weeks as a practicing Catholic.

So it was with the explicit purpose of having an orgasm that I took home *X-posure,* poured myself a glass of Chablis, dimmed the lights, slipped the tape into the VCR and myself into something more comfortable, and lit...goddammit!

Cut!

All I had in the apartment were those skinny, Chanukah candles, the result—along with a silver menorah—of a rare burst of sentimentality one holiday season back in Miami Beach when I decided to show Sam something about Chanukah. After we broke up and I moved north, I kept the menorah around for any future religious awakenings.

Providence, for here it was with *X-posure* cued and the room just crying for candle light. I retrieved it from the closet above the sink and set it on my side table, sticking a candle in every hole, and lighting them all with a bic lighter. Flame after flame fueled a mango-orange glow. The warm sheen enveloped my studio, as the candles roared irreverently against the black window pane. I pulled down the blinds, lest some zealot spot the sacred candelabra and bust in throwing stones.

I built a sanctuary of pillows on my bed and climbed aboard. Streams of light from the TV blending with my profane fire, I felt like a temple prostitute; numinous, on a quest for a new religion, seeking the wisdom of Silver Ray.

On screen: the scene.

Two women pretzeled in and out of each other's limbs; kissing, sucking, caressing. They were gorgeous, both with short, dark hair, nimble bodies, no implants, and even some cellulite, which I adored. Each was a mirror for the other. Together, they formed a kaleidoscope of feminine desire. I thought of Alexis watching me watch. Then she became Shade.

My right hand slipped inside the elastic band of my sweat pants.

My left hand held tight to the remote. I twirled my pubes between my fingers, spread my thighs further apart against the bed, let my fingers travel down and up so deep.

Meanwhile, on TV they were going at it furiously, one woman probing and pummeling the other with her fingers. Bring on the moan & groan track...*uh...uh...oh, god.* Silver Ray circles her clit with her middle finger, breathing bigtime, breathing in circles. She's going to come with them, she's sure. Come like she's wanted. Like she's needed. Into the fray, the fire, by the light of the glowing menorah, alongside this terbium orgy of tits and ass, she's pulsating to her toes, shucking and jiving like a mad bongo player...strumming on the old banjo, singing...

...Ringing!

A goddamn fire alarm chimed through the walls. *No, don't stop, don't stop...ignore it!* Another long, flat ring.

I jumped up and checked the menorah, which flickered innocently. The ringing continued. It was Yossi the doorman. I gave a breathless, "Hello?"

"Yes, it's Shade, she's here."

"What!"

"I send her to you."

The next few seconds were surreal. I stumbled up nervously, threw on a long-sleeved, black T-shirt, shut off the movie. My heart was beating as if I'd swallowed a double espresso with extra sugar, my thighs were damp inside my sweat pants. I felt slippery when I walked.

The doorbell rang. Before answering, I killed the fading glow of my early Chanukah celebration. I shouted, "Just a second!" and cursed myself for not spending the extra three hundred dollars a month for a one bedroom. In a studio you were on display like a caged animal. I opened the door and Shade barreled past me, a breeze of musk and sulfur. "How dare you not return my calls, I'm way too insecure for that shit—what's that smell?"

"Smell?" I asked, horrified.

"Something's burning." Her eyes roved left, right, bouncing from the silent images on the TV screen to the pile of pillows on my bed and landing finally on the smoking gun. "Is that a menorah?"

"Yeah," I shrugged, playing it oh-so-cool given the ubiquitous thumping in my temples. Her eyebrows lowered skeptically. "It's a candle holder, I didn't have any other candles."

"I thought you hated that new-age garbage." She stared at me, oddly. "What are you watching?"

"It's just background noise."

She took off her jacket and fell down on the couch with a loud, "Huh!" I sat on my bed perpendicular to her, watching as she quickly discovered the pile of videos Alexis had given me. She beamed her lowered eyebrows at me again. "Don't tell me, you've joined a Zionist sex cult."

"It's not what you think."

"I knew something was up, you haven't been you lately."

"I am the ghostwriter of Alexis Calyx."

"Great," she nodded. "Who's Alexis Calyx?"

Shade sat quietly as I explained just who Alexis was, describing with theatrical élan our first few meetings, playing up today's scene on the set. As it turned out, Shade knew of her; she'd once been to a feminist film festival where they banned one of Alexis' movies.

"Probably *X-posure,*" I threw out, suggesting intimate knowledge of the Alexis Calyx cannon. I wanted to appear hip, to talk about porn stars and sexual fantasies and Vaseline lenses. "There's some pretty hard-core fucking between women, even better than the boys do it."

Shade curled her upper lip and squinted.

"It goes beyond the usual girl-girl suck-fest."

"Girl-girl what fest?" She saw right through me. I shook my head and smiled dumbly. Shade said, "Okay, you fembot, who are you and what have you done with Rachel?"

"She went out for a quart of milk this morning, I haven't seen her since."

"And back in Miami I couldn't even get you to go to that stripper movie."

"You and your Hollywood porn."

"You know me, I'm a high-concept kind of girl."

I bit the inside of my lip, wishing for a bit of Silver Ray. She would know how to spin the situation, just as Alexis had twisted our conversation this afternoon. The best I could do was empty the rest of the wine into two glasses and sit down next to Shade on the couch. We laughed, bantering about the weather, the strike, other freelance possibilities, and just about everyone we knew. I would have forgotten how frustrated I'd been by her unexpected visit had I not found myself mesmerized by her pupils, the center of her gaze enlarged, encased in gold marbles; and her nose, her cheeks, her thick, fleshy lips jumped out at me, animated, as if they'd been properly lit for the first time.

Shade smiled, half-laughing. I folded my right leg further into my body and pulled my hair back. I would have sworn she was staring, too, although I was operating under the influence of pornography. They should put warning labels on those boxes. Like cigarettes. *Caution: Viewing may result in excessive fantasizing and skew sexual perceptions.*

"All right," I ventured. "What are you doing here?"

"I was trying to be mad at you. You're never around the picket line, so I'm stuck with the rest of those goombahs, and then you don't call me for three days, not even a message...you can't do that, Slivowitz. Nothing's stable anymore, I feel disconnected, like I'm all alone out here."

"What about Tina?" I said and immediately wished I hadn't. Saying her name out loud gave her too much importance.

"Oh, I can't talk to her. She's not about that." She stared at me so deeply that for the second time that day I felt as if I'd been stripped naked by the gaze of another woman. As much as I tried to look away, I kept coming back to her, smiling too much. Shade was so beautiful. Of course I'd always known that, but it had been more of a two-dimensional, fashion model sort of beauty. I felt as if in all the years we'd known each other I'd never really looked at her until now.

"You're making me nervous," she said. "The way you're looking at me, stop doing that."

"Doing what?"

"You know what." She rested her elbow on the couch and leaned her head against it. Our faces were almost touching.

"Are you really trying to seduce me, Slivowitz?"

"Yes," I said. Then, as if in slow motion, I watched myself bring my right hand to Shade's face. My fingertips burned against her chin. She shut her eyes, grazed her teeth against my fingers. I couldn't breathe, felt the world flash by in song lyrics. Birds do it, bees do it. Between the devil and the deep blue sea. Like a virgin.

I brought my lips to hers and we kissed a slow, soft kiss. My arms fell around her body and we were making out on my couch. The words reverberated in my head: *Shade and I are making out on my couch!* She twisted her hips slightly and pulled her head back. My lips slipped down to her neck. I kissed it. Still holding me, she whispered, "We can't do this."

"Yes, we can," I said, but I didn't want to talk. I kissed her again. This time, she grabbed a tight fist of my hair and pulled me close, kissing me longingly, lusciously. Her tongue traveled over my teeth, her lips riveting mine as if her own survival depended on it, and I remembered that Mark and Tessa hadn't kissed much. They were slamming and bamming like nobody's business, but without kisses? No wonder Tessa didn't come. At that moment I would have given anything to spend the rest of my life with Shade's tongue in my mouth.

But she pushed me away, stopping midscene. I had a newfound respect for Mark's frustration. This flicking on and off of desire was maddening.

I covered my face. My eyes felt dry, but I was afraid if I blinked I might start bawling. "I'm sorry," Shade said. She clasped her hands around mine and brought them to her lips. I remembered where my fingers had been earlier. Could she smell me? Taste me?

Without letting go, Shade brought our hands down to the couch. "Listen, we can't just kiss each other like that." I kept staring at our fingers, criss-crossed like a backgammon board. Connected. "Slivowitz, look at me." She lifted my chin. "I have real feelings here, this is no joke."

"I'm not joking, Shade."

"Okay, wait...look at it this way, I come in here and you're talking all of this sex talk and watching porno, and really, how do I know it's me you want? I could be anybody walking through that door."

"Oh, yeah, it was either you or the Dominos man. Luckily you showed up first."

"Don't start with your sarcasm, not with me."

I huffed, averting my eyes, thinking how much Shade reminded me of Alexis, both of them lecturing me, talking down to me. How was it that everyone but me seemed to know everything about my desire? If only I had some sense of what was going on behind Shade's stony face, beyond those eyes, which despite their discomfiting scrutiny made me want to hold her tight enough to cut off her circulation. Was I supposed to tell her about the porn? Tell her that, yes, just before she'd come, I was hot, I was horny, I was the phantom Silver Ray ready for anything and anyone, but in my Rachel Silver reality I wanted only Shade. I could tell her that I'd been thinking of her throughout *X-posure,* but I wasn't sure how she'd take it. If it were a compliment or an insult.

"This is too crazy," she said. And we carefully avoided each other's stares as we spoke a litany of innocuous little phrases until she angled over my shoulders to grab her jacket. I was flooded by waves of sadness and desolation; that left-alone-on-a-dark-desert-road feeling.

She stood up in front of me. I leaned back against the couch, hugging my knees into my chest. The lower corner of my left eye twitched.

"You're really leaving?"

"I can't stay, I'm scared."

"So am I."

"Please," she held out her hand. Begrudgingly, I took it and followed her to the door, more anxious than Tessa the porn star before her boy-girl debut. Whoever said sex was less pressured with women ought to have a lobotomy.

In the doorway, Shade put her arms around my shoulders, hugging me in the Alexis Calyx role. I moved in closer, slipping my hands inside her jacket, folding myself into her body, feeling through her sweater her shoulder blades, her ribs, the rough bumps of her spine, the hook of her hips. And her fingers were stroking me, her body on mine, our legs intertwined and breasts swept up against each other. How could she touch me like that and then leave?

"We'll talk tomorrow, okay?" she whispered, almost directly in my ear. I wanted to say don't go, but couldn't. Honestly, I wasn't sure which was more frightening: her rejecting me or changing her mind.

She pivoted on the lush carpet. I watched her glide down the hall, this electrified figure in my hospital-clean corridor. I wanted to run up behind her and take her to the ground in a girl-girl version of the *From Here to Eternity* wrestling scene. I wanted to say something important. But even more than that, I wanted her to come back here and tell me everything was going to be all right.

At the elevator bank, she turned and smiled. "By the way, you kiss good."

"Watch your language."

"The neighbors?"

"No, the grammar. You mean, well."

"No, I mean, *good.*" The elevator rang and Shade stepped inside. The doors whisked shut behind her. I felt dizzy, off-balance, and slid down against the molding in my doorway.

I'm not sure how long I was sitting there when I felt Freddy push her nose up against my face, meowing. She smelled like candle wax. Her face, I discovered, was covered with it: my little waxed pussy. What was it they said about you and curiosity, my furry friend? It hardly mattered, for I knew what they never said, that whatever doesn't kill you leaves you a complete and total mess.

Taking Care of Business

I squeezed my fingers around the telephone until my knuckles turned white. Listening to Shade's voice on the other end made my feet sweat. Several days had passed since we'd kissed, and I still couldn't talk to her without reliving the intensity with which my missionary lips had locked onto hers.

A cup of coffee teetered in between my thighs on the couch. Moted stripes of sun beamed through half-open blinds, double-exposing bars over my apartment like an illusive cage.

"I forgot to tell you, Alexis thinks I'm bisexual," I teased, the way only the telephone would allow. As if through the wires I had less at stake and could break through the hazy poles she'd erected between us. Alleviate the rejection I was feeling.

Shade laughed. "Bisexual?"

"Yup. But she says I'm probably man-primary. Apparently there's man-primary or woman-primary, she says it's about your emotional allegiances."

"What a visionary."

"Okay, forget it," I said.

"I'm sorry, it's just not that simple," Shade's voice cracked, and for one second, I thought she might be as frightened as I was. "You have no idea," she said. "Women will tear your heart out."

"Speak for yourself."

"Exactly, you're killing me."

"Is that why you're afraid to come near me? You froze up yesterday when I kissed you hello. On the cheek."

"For a smart girl, you're awfully dense."

"You say you're old enough to be my mother, you've got responsibilities." Those last words made me wince. Who was I to talk? My own "catch" quotient was down: no steady job, recently broke off an engagement, never been with a woman before. But Shade wasn't exactly stable.

"I can take you to a lesbian bar if you want," she said.

"I don't pick up men in bars, I'm not going to do it with women."

"Never let it be said I wasn't encouraging of your experimentation."

"I don't want an experiment, I want..."

"What? What is it you want?" she said, and I felt muzzled. I was valiant in my mind, I want to kiss you again, idiot. Instead I said, "You're driving me crazy."

"Then we're even."

"So now what?"

"Don't ask me," she sighed. "We crossed a line, anywhere we go it's trouble."

"Stop saying that. Why do you always say that?"

"Because I know. Now if you'll excuse me I have to go and get drunk before I remember I don't have anything else to do this afternoon."

I hung up feeling cast off. Jealous, too. Shade had become part of the strike, or at least one of the core journalists who'd been hanging around The Corral. Who knew the people she'd been cavorting with? The Tina Macadams of the world. Serves me right for abandoning my colleagues to shuttle back and forth between Alexis Calyx and Aunt Lorraine. I was on the outskirts; a journalist among journalists.

I walked to the sink determined to wash the few days worth of dirty dishes. Warm water trickled between my fingers. I remembered Shade's lips on my neck, her breath angling toward my ear. My hands found each other in between a few suds and I rubbed them together, slowly, feeling each finger the way Shade had touched them the other night. Pretending to be loved through my fingers. Hot water scalded my hands, my arms. The pounding in my chest expanded to my throat. I shut off the tap before picking up a single dish.I sat down on the couch, hiked my knees up next to me, thinking of Shade at home, maybe sipping from a 64-ounce Pepsi bottle or opening a can of tuna fish, careful not to let the oil drip between her fingers. Save those fingers for my touch. My lips. My tongue. I wanted her to bite me so hard she left teenage marks, then skim her tongue along the insides of my thighs until I screamed. My left nipple peaked through my T-shirt, sending adjectives rolling: hard, swollen, aching, empty.

I tore off the shirt and squeezed my breasts with both hands. As if I could wring my longing from them. My desire for a face so familiar I could barely remember it. I kicked my sweats to the floor and stepped in front of the full-length mirror, mindful of the savage glow in my eyes and Shade's voice: *You kiss good, Slivowitz.*

Naked, I pressed my palms against the mirror, its cool surface steaming at my touch. I gyrated my hips in a circle, swinging left and right like the Israeli dancers on public access TV. Whose body was this? Reeling in the rhythm of these hips...come swing with me and be my love...I caught a quick shadow of myself and had to fight another voice: *Look at you, the fat on your stomach jiggling, those awful asymmetrical nipples, that pubic sprawl on your thighs...who would want to touch you?*

Not Shade, not anyone; not even me.

I backed up into my dresser and scavenged my underwear drawer. Looking for a shield, a veil: the cover-up, please. I found the one black lace and silky bra I owned, a pair of shiny black underpants, and put them on along with my new platform boots that zipped up the inner calf, just like the ones Alexis wore. Prancing back and forth, I felt the power of my heels crush against the hard wood floor, the sweep of hair on my back.

Sexy as a character from an Alexis Calyx film, she was. The moment belonged to Silver Ray as she arched her back aware of the angle that kept her stomach taut for the camera. Her hand slipped into the swatch of satin between her legs. "My cunt is so wet!" she said.

And I laughed out loud at the ridiculous appeal of the words. Porno talk was generic, black letters on white packaging: napkins, soap, cereal, cunt. All object, no presentation. A wet cunt was what it was no matter how it got there. Last night it had been another Alexis Calyx video; today it was all me, or maybe Silver Ray, but it was for myself, or maybe for Shade, because she'd started it somehow, before everything became cloudy, except for my body in front of me.

I was a porn star in my mirror, here with my black bra and dirty words and thoughts of Shade holding me as I let myself go. The muscles in my legs contracted, my lips shook, and I closed my eyes to the breathing and moaning and screaming...*fuck me, make me come, oh yes!*

Generics. But they worked.

I lay on my mock-Oriental rug pondering another shower, my second today. I was breathing heavily, my throat parched and muscles jellied as if I'd been training all morning to run the New York City marathon, and I felt isolated. Lonesome in the quiet time, I got to my usual wondering about the philosophical nature of orgasms. If you come and nobody's there, did you come at all? And what if you could only come alone? Was the rest of it all rehearsal? The prelude to a life of solipsistic romance?

Not that I ever had any answers, but the questions themselves seemed less important than ever. There must be a joke about the journalist who stopped asking questions. I couldn't remember, I was too busy trying to forget.

Here is a truism I learned the very next day:

Nothing but nothing restores a girl's memory quicker than being with her family. With them, I was transported back to the turbulent climes of childhood, at speeds faster and more far-reaching than the Concord, which after all only goes two places. I'd moved to Miami to escape this proximity to my youth. "You'll come back, girls always do," Aunt Lorraine had said, and even then, green-eager at twenty-three years old, I knew she was right. Like Israel, we Slivowitzes clung to visions of eternal return.

I came back to Bay Ridge that November morning after spending more than an hour on the telephone with Mom the night before, trying to explain that yes, it was necessary for Dr. Milford P. Kaminsky to come to the house to see Aunt Lorraine and no, I hadn't intentionally planned for him to come on the day she'd set aside to start preparing Thanksgiving dinner. The holiday was a week away.

Yet, the moment I saw Hyman Hogan's Cadillac in front of the house and heard him scrambling to greet me at the door, I knew I was in for a difficult visit. Mom had summoned her protector. Who would help me? Our argument had distracted me so, I hadn't realized how afraid I was of this meeting with the good Doctor Suicide. I shivered, partially from the autumn wind, but also remembering the last time I'd seen Kaminsky. How I'd broken down like a cry baby. The girlie-girl running from her brothers.

Hyman Hogan yanked open the front door and, eyes twinkling, said: "Hey, Ray!"

"Hi, Hy!" I smiled and walked past him. Immediately, I noticed the hard-back chair rigged to a metal conveyor belt and attached to the banister of the staircase. The straps hanging from it made it look like an electric chair. I felt those straps tighten inside me, clamping my stomach.

Hy grabbed me by the elbow. "Glad you're here, Ray. Here, here, give me your coat, you can try out the chair. Rowdy had to be first already, but he scraped his hand against the wall, the moron. We got it from the magazine, the one doctors use. You should see what they got in there, it's unreal...what, what's the matter?"

My face must have betrayed the sickness I experienced upon viewing this anachronistic contraption, which reminded me of the movie *What Ever Happened To Baby Jane?* starring Joan Crawford and Bette Davis and seemed eerily apropos given the dynamics inside this Brooklyn brownstone. If I didn't know Hy, if I hadn't been aware of the benign spirit behind his thinning white hair and basset-hound face, I would have thought the chair a sick joke. As it was I just felt queasy.

Hy explained that he was always nervous watching Rowdy walk Aunt Lorraine up and down the stairs, so he thought the chair might ease her transport. "Go ahead, try it," he said. "Don't be scared, this thing could hold an elephant."

"Uh...maybe later," I demurred, saying I really should see Aunt Lorraine.

"She's asleep, been down for about an hour," he said. Our eyes met, and I knew he was about to offer an opinion. He had many opinions, most at odds with my own. I braced myself. "Say, Ray, it ain't right with this doctor. Lorraine's got goo-goo eyes from that lousy death movie. Why'd you do it?"

"I didn't do anything," I sighed, running my hand through my hair to cover my watery eyes, my unsteady chin. This man was not a member of our immediate family, he would not be allowed entry into Aunt Lorraine's hospital room should there be an emergency, and here he was ordering Baby Jane chairs and blaming me because Aunt Lorraine wanted to see Kaminsky. Mom had her old man brainwashed against me.

"The man's a bellyaching crackpot, a—"

"Look, I'm just doing what she wants, what she asked." My tone was as harsh as it had ever been with Hyman Hogan, and I feared becoming even more antagonistic. We stared at each other, adversaries in a war without words. I thought I smelled my breath mingling with his, breeding a new stench between us. If I tried to swallow I was afraid I might choke on it. Regurgitate the anger I was nursing.

"I guess it's nobody's fault really, just a tragedy all around," Hy said, shaking his head, though not exactly in contrition. It was more like the temporary stave of a good salesman. Before his son had taken over the family business, Hy had done his share of selling. Costume jewelry and plastic flowers. He'd been an ornamentalist.

"Mamma's in the kitchen, if you want to see her," he said.

I left him fiddling with the chair and went inside. Mom stood next to the kitchen sink. She was wearing her flowery satin housecoat, and her face was made up perfectly: blue shading beneath painted eyebrows, precise red lines on her lips, accent on the beauty mark above the left side of her mouth. I never understood the pains she took with her makeup when she had no intention of changing out of her bathrobe.

I kissed her powdered cheek and sat down at the kitchen table. We didn't talk, didn't have much to say without rekindling last night's argument, and I'd made a vow on the way out not to fight with her. She was breathing loudly, as usual, although her face looked almost serene, like a mother on television. I still kept a close watch on the knife she used to chop pecans for her Thanksgiving cranberry mold. It had always amazed me that my mother knew how to cook, a skill I was careful not to adopt by way of rebellion.

Mom was talking about the guy across the street who'd sold his brownstone to a family of Indians from India. I tuned out, letting my attention wander from the dingy cabinets to the sickly irises next to an old transistor radio on the windowsill. Was there anything new in this house? Mom called the Indians dot-heads. I didn't respond, just let the soft swish of the knife lull me into deep space.

"Rachel, stop it!" she screamed. I jumped up in my seat. Apparently I'd been shoving my fingernails into the gap between the formica tabletop and its metal siding. Not my fault the glue wasn't holding, again.

"Sorry," I said.

"You'll break the table yet," she said coolly, then turned back to her cutting. "Now, you're bringing the bread, right?"

"Bread?"

"Why do I bother...Thanksgiving? I'm saying it because last year the bread was a little stale, so if I were you I'd go somewhere else." She went on about the bread as if where I bought it would decide the entire fate of the holiday. The quickening chop of her knife was beginning to scare me. "Of course, I'm doing this all myself, nobody's coming in here helping me. You might try and help you know."

"I'll help you, I always do." I felt my pulse loosening a bit. "We have a whole week."

"I know, but I have to make sure everything's in place before I leave."

"Leave?"

"For Bermuda," she said as if I should have known.

"Bermuda?" I moved in closer to the cut and swish of her knife. "When are you going to Bermuda, why are you going to Bermuda?"

"Oh, I didn't tell you, we're going for the weekend, we leave tomorrow. I need a break, you know things haven't been easy for me lately."

"For you, what about Aunt Lorraine?" I paced, grabbed my hair. Mom pushed another pile of pecans closer to her knife with her shiny fingernails. Calm down, I thought. It's her life, she can go to Bermuda if she wants.

"That's what I'm saying, why I need some time away. For my health."

"You leave every weekend."

"Oh, some nerve you have; you, bringing death into this house. If you really wanted to help, you'd move back here and take care of Lorraine."

"She has a nurse, we're paying the nurse. You can't make me feel guilty for having a life. This isn't Victorian England."

"Then I won't feel guilty for taking a little weekend."

Her tempestuous chopping was making my head spin. I envisioned her slicing up her fingers then felt wicked for the thought. I counted backwards from ten, breathing deeply at the onset of each number, a technique I'd picked up in a day-long meditation workshop—two hundred bucks to learn how to count. Finally, Mom put down the knife, then brushed past me en route to the refrigerator. I turned my back and mumbled, "Go ahead, have your little weekend!"

"What?"

"Nothing, Mother." I was almost out of the kitchen, still huffing to myself. "Your whole life's been one long, little weekend."

"I heard that!"

She had to have the last word. I sunk into the sofa and stared out the living room window. My heart began to slow. A couple of kids raced bicycles down the street. The sky was overcast. Gloomy with ghosts. I'll bet the sun was shining in Bermuda. I longed for someone to whisk me away to Bermuda or back to my terrace in Miami with Shade lounging on a chaise of pink and yellow plastic in her bikini top and tight cut-off shorts. I realized my memory took a porno spin, but the day really existed.

I wore a conservative, one-piece Speedo and next to Shade felt fat, clunky, and prudish, watching her rub coconut oil into her caramel limbs. When I asked to borrow some she laughed.

"It's number four, black-girl shit. You need roots deep in the deserts of Africa."

"My people were slaves in the land of Egypt."

"Hah! Slaves of the Cossacks maybe," she smiled and pointed to her book, *Crime and Punishment.* She was the only person I knew—myself included—who still read serious books. They clashed with the pastel jogging suits and ice cold shopping malls. Miami was a land of recycled best-sellers. There were as many of them in the library at Grandma's nursing home as there were in an airport kiosk, the endless soft-cover spines cracked by tiny granules of sand.

"Who do you think crossed the Sinai?" I said. "Remember the Red Sea?"

"I remember Charlton Heston. The fascist."

"My father called him Charleston Heston."

"I like that, it makes him sound like an old southern queen," she said. "But you still need sunscreen, and none of that eight or fifteen nonsense, we're into the cancer hours."

Had it been a fantasy, I would have nixed the cancer and we would have made love as if it were a sex film: *Hot Terrace Babes.* Maybe we still could. Not satisfied merely imagining myself as Silver Ray, I had begun casting sex-extra roles to those around me. Why shouldn't my life be more like a porn film?

The doorbell rang. Answering it, I found Dr. Milford P. Kaminsky holding two plastic shopping bags, the weight of which seemed to push his frail body to its limits, as if he might fall over if you breathed on him too hard. One look at his sunken eyes and skeletal cheeks was all it took to eclipse my own problems.

Kaminsky handed me his tan parka, but insisted on keeping his shopping bags. I was hanging his coat in the front closet when I heard him say, "Hello."

I turned and saw him standing in the living room. Mom stood about fifteen feet from him at the dining room table, the knife at her side. She opened her mouth as if she were about to speak and collapsed to the floor, the metallic blade erect and glistening in her hand.

"Good Lord!" Kaminsky said, and dropping his bags rushed over to Mom. He removed the knife from her fingers and felt her pulse. "She's further along than—"

"Oh no, no. That's my mother," I said.

"This happens with some frequency then?"

I nodded and ran into the kitchen for the ammonia. No matter how many times Mom fainted, no matter how certain I was she'd brought it upon herself, I couldn't shake that initial flash of fear: What if it's real this time, if all along she'd been right? Even that day at the airport when I was leaving for Miami with her begging me not to go, I was at first terrified. She cried, grabbing at my coat, scratching my face. "Don't leave me!" she'd screamed.

I was sweating, weighed down by too many carry-ons, which I gripped tightly as Mom clung to my left arm. Trying to shake her off, I twisted my ankle. My sunglasses slipped down my nose. I stared at Aunt Lorraine, who tried to restrain Mom's arms with both hands. They were going to haul Mom off to Creedmore and I'd never get on that plane. The job, the apartment with the spiffy sundeck, the car I'd been waiting all my life to own would be history, and I would be stuck in Bay Ridge with my mother, who before that day had never shown so much interest in me or my life.

Aunt Lorraine held Mom back and turned to me. Her brow creased, her lips sewn with seriousness. "Rachel, go!" she said.

"Ungrateful, you!" Mom wailed. My eyes met Aunt Lorraine's who kept signaling me to leave, so I turned and took a few steps forward. Mom cried about losing her baby. I wanted to run to her and hug her, but we were never touchy-feely like that, and I resented her turning my departure into a scene at La Guardia airport. I peeked over my shoulder and saw her starting to teeter. She was fighting off Aunt Lorraine with her eyes open, but not fainting. On impulse I turned and walked back to them. Mom stared at me as if she were looking into her own grave. "I'm your mother...you...you're so selfish!" she sputtered, her face pink with frustration. I knew she was trying to faint, but couldn't. The way I sometimes tried too hard to come. Not to be undone by the physical boundaries of the act, however, she simply placed her hands in front of her, eased her body onto the airport floor, and lay down.

Aunt Lorraine and I hovered over her, watching dumbfoundedly as she bent her left elbow over her fluttering eyelids.

"Come on, Mom," I said. "This is ridiculous."

She didn't budge. Just lay awake, playing at fainting as people ambled toward us one-by-one, forming a crowd. Aunt Lorraine stared at me. "Go," she said again, and I didn't look back.

I found the ammonia under the sink, grabbed a roll of paper towels, and returned to Kaminsky. His fingers curled around Mom's limp wrist. I wondered if anyone had ever fainted in front of him before, had seen in him the face of death. I folded a paper towel in quarters, wet it with Ammonia, and leaned down next to Kaminsky.

"Here, let me," he said.

Handing Kaminsky the towel, I caught sight of Hy coming into the living room. He screamed: "STELLA!"

I bit my lip to keep from laughing, but the way he shouted her name...it wasn't her fault she was called Stella. Besides, this was serious. Mother has fainted—again. If I didn't get away I was certain to say something nasty. I counted backwards, as Kaminsky went about business, holding the towel to Mom's face as if he were a paramedic on a rescue show, pumping life back into Mom through white electrodes.

"Give me that!" Hy ripped the towel out of Kaminsky's hands, practically shoving the doctor out of the way, and I realized he might not be as benign as I'd thought.

"Hy!" I shouted. "Are you crazy?"

"Stella? Come now, doll?" Hy tapped Mom's cheek a few times with his fingers and then looked up at us. "Go away, would you?"

I apologized, touching Kaminsky's arm for emphasis. Mom's body stirred beneath her housecoat. She shook her head from side-to-side and said: "Monster!"

"Don't worry, I won't let him near you." Hy continued shooing us away.

I led Kaminsky through the living room as Mom's screaming echoed. We came to the stairs with that damn Baby Jane chair, and I tried to pretend it was normal to have a wooden chair strapped to a dolly on the staircase by suggesting that we walk single file next to it. I started feeling slightly ghoulish myself with Kaminsky rustling his plastic bags behind me, making me think of candelabra, blood-sucking vampires, and loud, fearful screams. Like Mom's.

As if that weren't enough, we found Aunt Lorraine asleep with an Alexis Calyx movie playing on her giant television set. We were so alike in temperament, my old aunt and I. I knew she'd be curious about the videos, and remembering what they'd been doing to me, I became embarrassed for her. She herself was less stressed about the subject matter, leaving those tapes running continuously like a peep-show booth.

I shut off the TV and offered Kaminsky a chair. Either he hadn't noticed the movie or he was pretending not to, just as he'd followed my lead with the Baby Jane chair, and with Mom. Besides, in his circles, he must have seen things stranger than a dying woman who'd developed a taste for come shots and daisy chains.

I leaned over and rubbed her arm. "Aunt Lorraine?"

"Honey," she opened her eyes and slowly moved her head to the side, turtlelike, as if her neck were a periscope. "Oh, and Milford, you made it! You don't look a thing like I pictured."

"Most people tell me the opposite."

"So how was your trip?"

"Fine."

"You took the D train?"

"No, I have the car," Kaminsky said. "There was hardly any traffic, I made it in less than an hour."

Within minutes, they were laughing and talking like old friends, obviously continuing one of the numerous telephone conversations they'd had in the past few weeks. They didn't need me, and hardly noticed when I excused myself to go downstairs and check on Mom, who was sipping from a ceramic cup at the kitchen table with Hy stroking her arm and whispering to her as the coffee pot burped in the background. For the first time in a while, Mom looked settled. I suppose Hy soothed her, made her world more manageable, just as Kaminsky would do for Aunt Lorraine.

I sat down on the steps next to the empty Baby Jane chair, trying to remember the last time I felt settled. Certainly not with Sam in Miami, and never with Ethan, and not even with Jeremy, my.... I never knew what to call him, my journalism professor at Brooklyn

College. In the beginning he told me he'd been sent to guard me from the world, and thinking back to the night Dad sat on my bed to shield me from Neil, I felt comforted. Like I'd found home. As time went on I realized Jeremy was mostly protective of our secrecy so his friends and colleagues wouldn't realize he was screwing a student. At least he'd phoned Columbia for me. All told, I traded my virginity for a scholarship to journalism school.

I never missed him. Never missed any of them once they were gone. It was Alexis' voice I heard next: *Rachel, are you a lesbian?* Again I ignored the question, tired as I was of these people battling for air-time in my mind.

The front door clicked open and in walked Rowdy. His face was stubbled, and he wore a torn flight jacket over khaki pants a few sizes too big for him. I used to think he might be gay. Back when I was a teenager and he had a girlfriend, a hairdresser named Betty. Betty had auburn curls and thick fingers that dwarfed my hand when she took it in hers and, in her curbside drawl, said: "Hello, Rachel, darling." After she and Rowdy broke up, Neil told me she used to be a man. "Sick fuck cuts it off and then she's hot stuff, too good for our brother." Neil laughed in that eerie way I never quite heard, but felt in the small of my back. "Serves him right the fucking faggot." As far as I know that was the last relationship Rowdy ever had; nobody ever mentioned it.

Rowdy leaned his elbow against the banister and shook a cigarette from a package crushed so badly I couldn't recognize the brand. They were simply cigarettes: generics. He lit up and inhaled deeply, opening the screen door to toss the match outside. Cigarette smoke blended with the scent of wet leaves.

"You like that asparagus in the can?" he said.

"Sure."

"It's on sale, three for two by Waldbaums. They let you take three at a time, but I go back to a different cashier." He smiled as if he'd discovered a secret stash of gold, then pulled a few cans out of a paper bag. "Here, take a few with you."

"Thanks," I said.

Rowdy sat down in the doorway, propping the screen door open with his right foot. His vinyl athletic shoes had no laces, his feet had grown too wide for them from the phlebitis, and his experimentation with the Baby Jane chair had left a huge raspberry on his left hand, like the ones he used to give me whenever we played Knuckles. The card game was a lot like Spit. "One, two, three, Go!" we screamed as our hands flipped quickly the diamonds, clubs, hearts, and spades and the higher number gobbled up the pile, winning that round. When the cards were gone and winner had taken all, the loser shuffled and whatever number was drawn was the number of times the winner got to scrape the deck over the loser's knuckles. I never won.

Odd, how the menacing forces of youth have a way of weeding themselves out in adulthood, Rowdy mutating from a teenager who'd ripped the skin from my knuckles to this off-kiltered man with the huge raspberry and swollen feet, who might be gay and had a hard time remembering anything that wasn't written on a coupon insert. "Business sucks," he said, and I was afraid of the business he was up to these days. "Used to be a guy could make a buck around here before the tree-lovers took down the recycling business. They don't know all they're helping is the mafia."

"Looks like you need a new line of work," I said, remembering the fights he and Mom used to have over the hundreds of cans and bottles he'd collected from the streets, some bought at a cut rate from people more indigent than himself, the bottom of the bottom-feeders. He would clean and sort the stash, then return them to the supermarket for deposit money.

"Funny you say it." He dragged from his cigarette and craned his neck sideways to look at me. "Maybe you can help."

"Me?"

"Yeah, you and your porno friends. I know a lot of people around who'd be interested in what they got. There's only one store in the neighborhood that sells porno."

I stared at him thinking Alexis would be mortified. Her videos might occupy the same cosmic shelf space as *Anal Beach Party* or *Come With The Wind,* but she prided herself on getting them into feminist bookstores as well. She would not appreciate Rowdy peddling them on the street alongside the used appliances, old magazines, and grainy copies of Hollywood movies shot from the back row of a theater. But I couldn't tell that to Rowdy. Why disappoint his fantasies of making his way, of becoming the person who always seemed to be skipping just a beat ahead?

No matter how many times I convinced myself I was adopted, that I shared nothing with my brothers but the occasional meal and, when we were growing up, a bathroom, our kinetic links came in subtle moments, like the spot-light recognition of nostrils too large or a sunken earlobe. Like now.

I wondered if Rowdy had ever felt settled; with Betty, perhaps? He stared at me dumbly, saliva pooling inside of his lower lip. He was about the same age as Alexis Calyx, yet he looked at least a decade older. I was suddenly frightened for him. "I guess I can talk to Alexis," I told him, knowing that I wouldn't.

"Got to get something going, man," he nodded.

"I can't promise anything."

He waved his hand dismissively as if he'd grown impatient with our conversation and lit another cigarette. I felt the wind creep up my spine. Night was descending on Bay Ridge.

I was late to meet Alexis Calyx. Never in my life had I been so constantly running late. To arrive early was a journalist's trick: you never knew what you might catch a person doing before they were expecting you. It could make for great color.

Alexis waved me inside her office. There was a man sitting in one of the leopard skin chairs across from her desk. He turned his head, and I recognized him immediately. Despite the few gray twists in his dark brown hair, the fuller cheeks and deeper dimpling of his chin, Robbie Rod looked the same as I remembered him from *Sensurround.* All swarthy and seductive. And I couldn't forget those eyes, the dark brown irises swimming in sad, luminous circles. In person, his eyes were even more inviting, if not downright humanizing. Eyes that made me wonder why he'd never pursued a legitimate acting career until I recalled his other stellar attribute, careful not to let my gaze wander where it shouldn't.

"This is Rachel Silver, my ghostwriter," Alexis said.

"Ah, the new scribbler," he said and turned to Alexis. "This one looks like you, maybe she'll last."

"This one?" I said, taking the empty seat next to him. He smelled clean, as if he'd just showered and shaved. "Okay, just how many were there?"

Alexis, grimacing nervously, promised me the number wasn't important, although I felt my balance shifting as this man jabbed at the precarious fulcrum of my employment. "Let's see," he counted on his fingers. "There was the star-fucker, the manic-depressive, the closet Christian..." As he spoke, I stared at his fingers—nails evenly filed, cuticles trimmed, a thin silver and turquoise ring on the fourth finger of his right hand, they seemed of a different class than the rest of his body, as if they should have accompanied a double-breasted suit instead of crisp black jeans and Italian loafers. The fingers of a banker or company president. Fingers that inspired trust. I always studied men's fingers, even before I moved in with Sam and every night held his thin hand wondering how many vaginas it had explored that day. His fingers said he was a gynecologist right down to their chalky tips. One might have expected the same of a porn star, hands that betrayed his profession, but this man sitting next to me, this legend of the stroke houses, his fingers were elegant and omniscient. His pinkie sprang back to join the rest of its clan as he pinpricked Alexis. "We wouldn't want to forget your sister," he said. "Your own flesh and blood."

"You made your point," Alexis said.

"Right, she only lasted a week," he said, turning to me. "Forget the sister."

I nodded okay. There was too much tension in the room for clever repartee. Besides, I couldn't believe what he'd mapped out on his feelers: I was the fourth ghostwriter. Fifth if you included the sister.

Alexis sighed as if she'd been through this performance one time too many. She raised her eyebrows at me. "Need I introduce the bastard sitting next to you?"

"Robbie Rod," I blurted, embarrassed by my own enthusiasm. I tried to cover by telling him I liked his work, which made me sound even more idiotic. My head played Shade's voice: *Nice going,*

Slivowitz. He probably thinks you're a true-blue sycophant like the last ghostwriter, or another manic-depressive, a closet Christian—I had gone to the confession booth as a child—or just another lonely woman in New York besieged by biological clocks and beauty myths.

"Thanks, but I'm not your guy," Robbie Rod said. His face and his voice were equally flat, emotionless, and firm, as if he were a bodyguard or, more precisely, an actor playing a bodyguard. I sensed he was too cunning to spend his life protecting anybody but himself. "Poor boy put a semi to his head a couple years back," he said. "Real catastrophe."

"Must be tough when the fan mail stops," Alexis furrowed her brow at him.

"Actually it was his ex-wife who did him in."

Alexis grunted as if this man's presence had stalled her verbiage. That was a first. She grabbed a long, black raincoat from the rack behind her chair. "You ready?" she asked. I nodded.

"Wait, where are you two going?" Robbie Rod or whomever he was now said.

"Out."

He held out his palms. "Excuse me, but?"

"What do you think, Rachel, shall we take the poor man to dinner?"

They both stared at me. "Um...sure."

"All right, I'll go along if you want, but I'm buying," he said.

"Oh, okay," Alexis mocked his tough-guy posture, the way he threw his shoulders back to make them look bigger. I watched him stretch his arms into a worn leather jacket, looking normal enough for a dead icon.

Outside, the streets were strangely quiet, blue with the tease of evening. I had the sensation of walking through a dream where the landscape looks familiar but isn't, where people seem to speak your language but don't. We floated a few blocks to a small Korean restaurant and were ushered to a table next to the front window. I was convinced our hostess had placed us there deliberately. To be seen. And these retired porn stars still cut a stunning duo, both so tall and well-designed, as if they'd been eugenically cultured with a flair. Around them I felt short and dumpy.

Another stylish couple at the next table kept looking over at us and whispering to each other. Probably they recognized one or both of my celebrated companions. Maybe they knew enough industry scuttlebutt to wonder what business had brought these two together tonight. If Alexis were wooing her famous ex-husband for a movie. Or could there be a reconciliation brewing? And was I one of their lawyers? The kid sister? A new talent ripe for the plucking? Whatever their confidential murmurs, I liked seeing myself through the eyes of these strangers. They knew nothing about me, except that based on the company I kept, I must be hip, liberated, and maybe even a bit kinky.

Three large bottles of beer arrived at our table, curtailing visions of my own kinkiness, but not before I'd resolved to buy myself a leather object that couldn't be found in a department store. Alexis smiled at the waiter. Robbie Rod looked bored. The three of us were silent as the waiter filled each of our glasses, leaving enough space on top for three zealous bursts of foam.

"I'm still pissed about this Claire thing," said Robbie Rod, his tone a melange of anger and exasperation, his pose pure gadfly. I watched his fingers curl around the stem of his beer glass.

"And it's still none of your business," Alexis said. "You're the one who bowed out."

"My money's in this thing."

"No strings, remember?"

"It's not even like she's headlining anymore."

"She's an artist."

"Says who?"

"Everyone. She gets grants all the time."

"For screaming obscenities in a refurbished bath house; what a racket," he said so calmly I wondered if he had a pulse. "This is why I hate New York, everybody's an artist. You take a shit in public, and as long as you serve wine, it's art."

I couldn't help laughing, which incurred a malevolent side-glance from Alexis. But he was right, this woman didn't sound like an artist.

"You think he's funny?" Alexis turned to me.

I shrugged, smiled weakly.

"As if that's not the easiest criticism...ugh," Alexis sighed. I stared at the bubbles in my beer glass. Appetizers of crab salad and oily spring rolls arrived at our table, but nobody touched them. I wished they would put a fork in the conversation and settle into the meal.

"She can't act," he said.

"Who cares? She's French," Alexis said as if that made all the difference. I thought of French kisses, French ticklers, French cuffs...the Moulin-Rougue and Catherine Deneuve. She had him there: being French was sexy.

"So you got a frog performance artist in a porn film, what a coup." He lifted a spring roll with his thumb and forefinger and dropped it on his plate, wincing, "Ah, mother!"

Alexis dipped her chopsticks into the crab salad. I reached for a spring roll with my fork and started eating immediately. Though thankful for the activity, I was careful not to eat too much or too fast. A woman of normal appetite, I imagined him noting, no sadomasochistic relationships with food.

"If you've got problems with my actors, make your own damn movie," Alexis said.

"How can I when you're sucking up all my funding?"

"It's not my fault you gave up," she said, and they were back in the ring. My temples pounded, the back of my neck felt like a rubber band, stretching. As much as I was embarrassed watching Alexis thrown on the defensive, I couldn't help being fascinated by this man who stood up to her. My allegiances had become more tenuous. I was fourth, after all—fifth if you included the sister.

As their argument progressed, I learned that Claire Blue was one of the attractive brunettes from *X-posure.* Alexis loved her; Robbie Rod hated her. It had something to do with the last time they'd worked together. He did fixate on the word bitch, just as much as he harped about being the one who'd hooked up the financing for *One in the Hand, Two in the Bush.* Alexis' chin dropped. She said he and his people were minimally involved. He begged to differ. And like that, they continued.

Luckily, I had to concentrate on rolling strips of beef and onions and beans and peppers into a big leaf of Romaine lettuce without making too much of a mess. When my attempts became futile, but no more than theirs, I ordered another beer, which slackened the rubber band in my neck. I listened to the two of them, mesmerized by their voices, captivated by the exaggerated wrinkling and cracking of these faces, whose hostile stares belied two people who might actually like each other. I wondered how often they spoke on the telephone, if he stayed in her apartment when he was in town, if they still had sex

By the time the busboy cleared our plates, the stylish couple at the next table, and most of the people in the restaurant for that matter, had disappeared. The waiter brought us three decafs. Alexis tapped his arm, "Do you have anything boozy? Something sweet?"

"Rice wine," he said.

"Oh no, you know, Sambuca? Goldschlager?"

"Rice wine."

"Peppermint Schnapps...no? Okay, a glass of rice wine, please," she smiled politely, then excused herself to go to ladies room, leaving me alone with Robbie Rod just when the conversation seemed to be returning to familiar ground. I took the soiled paper napkin from my lap and started shredding it on the tabletop.

"She's got no business sense," this man sitting across from me shrugged, his face lifeless and incomprehensible. I thought of Rowdy talking earlier about business, how his cheeks had dropped as if they'd lost their muscle, how his eyes had tinted with sorrow. I started feeling sentimental and hated myself, then I hated this man with his cool confidence, his big business and big dick.

"You think I'm an asshole," he said.

"No," I said seriously, as if I were being questioned for jury selection. He nodded his head back and forth, smiled. I leaned my chin against my fist. "Not really."

He sucked his tongue against his teeth and nodded. "I'm just a pragmatist. Alexis may think recognition from a bunch of cellophane skins makes her an artist, but I know better; the only art in this world is making money."

"Jesus, you're more cynical than I am."

"My guess is you're no cynic at all, Silver."

"What? What did you call me?" I was stunned. In his eyes, I saw myself writhing in the mirror. Not Silver Ray, but the slightly overweight, hips-too-big, tits-too-small Rachel Silver, exposed. The back of my neck felt hot, and I got a warm whiff of my pussy.

"Isn't that the way journalists do it?" he said. "Last names only."

"Oh." I giggled self-consciously, and he put his right hand to his cheek as if he were talking on a mobile phone. "Johnson, Silver here, the president is dead. His guts smeared all over my notebook, it's fantastic."

"Okay, I can start stereotyping porn stars any time now, Robbie Rod." The truth was I couldn't think of anything to say that didn't involve his penis. Under no circumstance would I let this conversation become sexual.

"I told you Robbie Rod is no longer with us." He crossed his arms in front of him as if he were the first person ever to perform the tired gesture. Funny thing was, it worked for him. He fit that tightly in his own skin.

"Right, I forgot, everyone's dead with you. Whatever you say, RR." I looked away. I didn't want him to see how nervous he was making me. I started pushing my napkin shreds into a neat pile, then remembered Mom telling me not to play with objects on the dinner table. The moments when propriety struck her often amazed me. She could pretend to faint in the middle of a crowded airport, but I couldn't touch the leftover food on my plate when we were home alone.

I looked up and RR was staring at me. I wondered if he too thought I had no class, playing with napkin shavings as I was. Alexis would never tear into a napkin.

"Listen, I mourned," he said.

"You what?" I cocked my head, journalistically.

"It's not easy losing a legend, but you move on. Sort of like how video killed the radio star."

"I think you need to get out more."

"I get out too much." He tilted his head as if the cameras were rolling, and I thought, what a smug, arrogant slob. If only I could stop flirting with him.

I smiled despite myself. "You talk like a porn film."

"Doesn't everyone?" he said, and our eyes met, long enough for my neck to flush, long enough that I was sure he could see Silver Ray coming into her own.

She wanted me to break rules and destroy confidences, cross double yellow lines and talk generic porno talk as if I'd invented the words myself. But not here, with him, in a Korean restaurant. I peeked down at my pile of napkin strips, empty glasses greased with three sets of lip prints, the lazy glimmer of a wick buried to its head in liquified wax. You couldn't get more postprandial, and this, for some reason, made me antsy. I stuck the tip of my index finger into the candle and felt the heat shoot up my arm. Shuddering, I pulled it away. He laughed, and we stared at my finger in its cloudy white thimble until Alexis returned, and I quickly hid my hand underneath the table. I spent the rest of the meal playing with the wax on my finger.

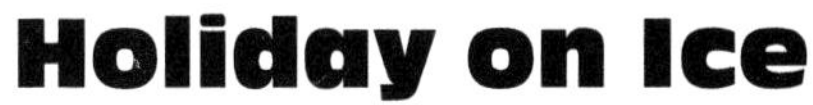
Holiday on Ice

Mom set down the holiday china and crystal as I followed with Grandma's silverware. At the head of the table she stopped and twirled around to face me, a curious glint in her eyes. Hugging a couple of plates to her stomach, she burst into song: "*I'm as corny as Kansas in August...ya, da, da, ya, da, da, Fourth of July.*"

I dropped a few forks and stood frozen, afraid she might slip off to Bali-Hi. I wondered if Hy knew we could be dining in the South Pacific. But Mom simply pirouetted backwards and resumed her table setting, singing, "*I'm in love, I'm in love, I'm in love, I'm in love....*"

It had been a while since I'd been ambushed by her off-key crooning. Growing up, she used to sing along with the albums and address us by characters' names as if we were all part of the show. So many times we'd heard how before she met Dad she'd been headed for Broadway, yet as far as I knew the closest she'd come was once auditioning for a regional production of *Oklahoma.* And her knowledge of musicals curtailed in the mid-seventies, after she'd seen *A Chorus Line.* That was her show. She'd taken me to see it twice. Both times we stood for hours at the half-price ticket line and then stuffed ourselves silly with shrimp at Beefsteak Charlie's. By the time we got to the theater I was so tired I slept through both performances, but remember once having to pee and opening my eyes to actors singing about breast implants. I leaned my body closer to

Mom's and whispered, "Ma, I have to—" "Uh, Rachel, your breath stinks." She shooed me away without taking her eyes from the stage. I drifted back to sleep with my hand holding my crotch and dreams of mint chewing gum.

"Oh, I'm really in love again," Mom said. She grabbed my upper arms and I shivered, forced a smile.

"I'm happy for you."

"And Hy is a wonderful guy. So romantic."

Her grip on my arms felt stifling, more like a choreographed move than a show of affection. Her fingers smelled like turkey guts. I had to pull away.

She followed me back into the kitchen and yanked open the oven. The candied scent of sweet potatoes sailed through the kitchen. One hand encased in an oven mitt, Mom slid out the tray and like a surgeon inspected the bird. "Rachel, give me that thingy, would you?"

I handed her the baster, watched her suck up the juices puddled alongside of the turkey and release the liquid over its crisp brown skin. "I was thinking this might be the last holiday, you know, with Aunt Lorraine," I said.

"Yes, but we have Hy and his family now." She brushed off my feelings faster than the juices trickled down the sides of that damn bird. It took all I had to overlook her selfishness. I thought of Aunt Lorraine, what she might wear today to cover her bald head.

"Don't you see we're gonna be a whole family again?" Mom said. "I even tried to get Neil and some woman, she sounded like a real you-know-what. She told me not to call so much, but we don't know her, who is she?"

"He lives with her, I think it's her house." Neil had told me he was moving in with his girlfriend the last time he called me from Vegas. I was still living in Miami then. He asked me for five hundred dollars, which I sent to him, as I'd done sporadically over the years. I would do whatever I could to support his life away from mine.

"Neil's a jerk, always was."

"So he's excused from seeing his mother?" she said, still basting. "Oh, by the way, there's something for you there, in the little brown bag." I opened it and pulled out a wooden pop-gun, painted with green and yellow leaves and a palm tree on each side of the handle. The word BERMUDA was scrawled in black letters on top. A piece of cork hung from a string attached to the handle.

"Mother, you bought me a weapon." I slammed the handle forward and the cork went flying: pop! Just like a bottle of wine.

"Isn't that the best?" Mom laughed. "We had such a time down there. One night we were out on the beach, you could see a million stars, it was so clear, like a painting." I loaded up, cocked the handle of my toy gun back and forth like a saw, gearing up for another pop. "So Hy tells me all those stars are nothing compared to my eyes; my eyes sparkle like diamonds, he says. And he should know, he's in jewels."

"I thought his jewels were fake." I popped the gun. The airy bang left me feeling satisfied, justified.

"Oh, you're the big jewelry expert now," Mom said. She stuck a fork in between the turkey's legs to taste the stuffing, and I couldn't help but think of the obligatory spread-eagled porn star. I had a vision of Mom with her legs spread and Hy wriggling on top of her, coming like a pop-gun...*isn't that the best?*

I put down the toy gun.

"I'm just saying how sweet a man he is," Mom said. "And I'm getting on with things, that's more than you can say."

"What is that supposed to mean?"

She pushed the turkey back into the oven, slamming the door behind it. "Just the other day I was telling Hy, I'm worried about Rachel...you're turning into one of those snot-faced Manhattan girls." Mom shook her head at me. "You think you're so smart, but look, even Neil's got a live-in. Before you know it you'll be forty and then fifty and you'll be too set in your ways. You'll end up like Lorraine, a spinster. And look what happened to her."

"You're saying if I don't get married I'll get breast cancer?"

"Yes! There are studies, you write articles, but do you ever read them? They say women without children have more trouble because you're supposed to have children. It unlocks your hormones."

That Aunt Lorraine never married had always irked Mom; that I, having called off one wedding already, was headed in the same direction was her filial nightmare. Yet as Mom spoke, I realized that from the day Sam and I registered at Burdines, I knew we would never make it to the pulpit. But after a year of his proposals I was tired of him and everyone else asking, when are you getting married? I was also convinced I'd contracted a Yuppie disease. Worn down from workaday ailments, the diarrhea, the allergies, the half-moons under my eyes, I looked and felt a decade older than my twenty-nine years and started seeing myself in equations of security: Mrs. Anglo Saxon, Mrs. Miami Coop, Mrs. Gynecologist, a baby-maker for her babyman, who spent his days sticking his hands up women's pussies and his nights coming home reeking of cunty rubber gloves. No surprise my vagina never worked anywhere near him. Even after he'd put me on the Kegel regimen: fifty a day, usually in my jeep driving to and from work. Sam was hopeful. Thinking it was about needing exercise. Thinking it was about needing therapy. Thinking it was about orgasms. The truth was that despite all the security in the world, I didn't want to be his wife. Or anybody's. I had a marriage disease. The day Sam and I broke up I felt as if I'd stepped outside for the first time after a three-year flu. I tossed out the skin pills, the snot pills, the shit pills, the nerve pills.

Mom had been afraid for me since I broke off my engagement. Her eyes blazed a history of fears: isolation, loneliness, displacement, homelessness. If only I could tell her I shared them, too. Just as I still believed in love, still longed for someone to whisper to me when insomnia swooped in, someone who knew touching was better than coming, but those desires seemed antithetical to finding myself on a beach with a know-it-all-man telling me my eyes were like diamonds, dialogue even too banal for a porn film. Dialogue that suited mother's cant.

"You have to start facing reality," she was saying, "haven't you heard about the chances of finding a husband after thirty?"

I broke her mid-monologue. "Ma, enough already. Don't you think I worry about this? I'm not a total flake."

She tipped her head sideways as if the new angle might help her decipher whether I was lying or not. "Something is different," she said.

"Everything's different, even my toothpaste."

"Don't be smart."

We stood eye-to-eye. She was breathing loudly, squeaking through her nose. A shylock nose with big pores, a gift I'd inherited as well. I wanted her to hug me, to touch me like a fantasy mother without an agenda. But neither one of us moved.

"And don't you start with any of that porno stuff either, Hy is a nice man."

"What do you think I am?" My anger rose with her amplified snorting. On occasion I remember wanting to plug up her nose with tissues. I could be as repulsed by her as she'd been by my adolescent breath.

"Finish the vegetables, would you?" she snorted and exited the kitchen.

I could hear her singing the Kansas in August song, which gnarled my stomach as I peeled and cut the carrots, then ran a couple of bell peppers under the tap. They looked as if they'd been tie-dyed in streaks of red and yellow and green: hippie vegetables. I held one in each hand, like breasts. Thoughts of Shade flooded in with the streaming water.

We'd been having coffee at The Movie House, watching as the coupled and contented tourists passed, when on impulse I asked her to come for Thanksgiving. She smiled. "Sure, why not?" My muscles tensed imagining myself telling Mom I was bringing a friend. The word friend had never felt so nuanced, as if it had fallen under the dominion of my tongue. I was afraid I couldn't say it with the neutrality that being with my family demanded.

My feelings were at day's end, moot. Shade called at eleven. "Actually, I don't think I can deal with your racist, homophobic family."

"Neither can I." I laughed it off. But there I was left holding my crotch again, a rejection I could have surpassed had Shade not called back the next day to tell me she'd been up all night tossing it over, and she did want to come after all. Then, a few hours later, she'd changed her mind again, and for the next five days we played a game of bumper cars, slamming into each other and pulling away, until my stomach soured and my nerves were raw. I started looking to that jerk Robbie Rod for comic relief.

The tension of the last few days returned as I slid the knife through each of the psychedelic peppers, and with shaky fingers scooped out the white seeds and threw them in the garbage. By the time Shade had given me her final no, I was so enervated I wasn't even relieved the indecision was finally over. Now, I wished she'd come. I wanted to let my knee bump up against hers underneath the dinner table, or feel her comfort me with a hand on my thigh so I could make it through this Thanksgiving, even if it was Aunt Lorraine's last. The way we were going, though, Shade would probably pull back too soon, leaving me despondent and morose, isolated among my own people.

I sliced the peppers into narrow sections like arthritic fingers, divided them in two piles, then fit them in between the carrots, celery stalks, cucumber slices, and tiny cauliflower heads already on the lazy Susan. I lifted the tray and walked into the living room. Hy and his family were sitting with Rowdy.

"Hey, Ray!"

"Hi, Hy!" He was wearing suspenders with little turkeys on them. "Nice suspenders."

"Thanks, got them in Singapore."

"Tell me what the damn chinks know about turkeys," Rowdy laughed. He was sitting on the windowsill, smiling at passing cars like a circus clown who'd lost his troop. "You don't see no Turkey Chow Mein, Hy. Know what I'm saying? No Moo Shu Turkey."

Hy ignored him in favor of introducing me to his son and daughter-in-law, Evan and Ellen. I went to shake their hands but had a tray full of vegetables and nowhere to put them, since the coffee table was filled with bowls of popcorn.

"What's this?" I adopted Mom's happy-go-lucky, musical theater posturing. In recent years I'd honed a friendly Q&A mode for the holidays, as if my family were part of an ongoing human interest story. Asking questions worked better than saying, for instance, Get these dirty Tupperware bowls off the coffee table, Rowdy, you freak.

"It's cool, ay?" he said. "Tony gave me a whole bag, from the movie theater." He pointed his thumb to a green Hefty bag near the front door.

"I love movie popcorn," Evan said, grabbing a handful and popping it into his mouth. It didn't have a healthy crunch, sounded like he was chewing on styrofoam. But Evan, his right cheek bulging, said it was delicious. He had inherited Hy's droopy features, although his thick brown mustache and tortoise-shell glasses made his face seem wider. He was dressed like a manager on his day off: knit sweater with an Oxford shirt beneath it and tan corduroys. His wife Ellen wore a forest green pants suit and humongous gold hoops in her ears, a fringe benefit of working in the family jewel business. She smiled and bent down to help me clear the popcorn as if she were used to accommodating people.

"Hey, don't take it all," Rowdy said.

"We can't just serve popcorn, much as we'd like to," I said.

He winced.

"We'll just shuffle things around a little," Ellen said. She smiled kindly at my brother, the way people who didn't know him usually did at first. Next came the desire to help him. He had the kind of look that inspired the need to feed him, clothe him, bathe him, and then send him away. A Hefty bag full of popcorn was loose change. I'd seen him come home once with a leather jacket, fresh lobster, and some hand-me-down electronic equipment; just that morning he showed me a clunky old videocassette recorder a guy at the supermarket had given him the week before. He said he'd been videotaping Aunt Lorraine. Kaminsky'd suggested it, and Rowdy figured he could make a *Docudeath* tape as good as anyone.

Amateur, I thought.

Like the amateur porn Alexis railed against. The idea was too populist for her: if people started making their own videos, then her images decreased in value. Alexis had that Marxian sense of exploitation common to many who made a living in the skin trade.

Ellen and I fit the vegetables, a cheese board, and basket of crackers on the table and left room for two bowls of popcorn. Rowdy planted the rest of the bowls throughout the living room, setting them on shelves and side tables, and then started fiddling with his video camera. He lifted it to his face and commanded us to smile.

Still in Q&A mode, I asked Evan and Ellen how they met as Rowdy haunted to and fro with the camera at his face.

"I work for them," Ellen said.

"You should see her, Ray," Hy said. "Got sales in the blood. She was employee of the month, not once or twice, six times in a row. Even sold to the Army. The Army, can you believe it? What soldiers need with satin flowers? Unreal."

"She asked how we met, Dad, not for a resume," Evan said. He picked up the conversation from there, taking me from the first time he saw Ellen in the office to the day just last week, when after months of searching for a home in New Jersey, they'd closed the deal on a house in Upper Montclair near Ellen's parents.

"Say that again," Rowdy said. Evan squinted at him, obviously perplexed. "Come on, come on, I had my hand on the wrong side, just say what you said."

"The same thing?"

"What, you got wax in your head or something? Yeah."

Evan repeated the story of their olympiad search for the perfect house, hardly conscious that it was the second telling. Rowdy held tightly to the camera, occasionally slipping his left hand down to scratch his balls. I remembered first Alexis the other day calling her camera the best dildo she ever had, and then my father years ago posing us in front of his 8 x 10 camera, picking at his dick as he ordered us to wet our lips for the camera.

We were a clan of voyeurs, devouring newsreels and newspapers, musicals, movies, weekly magazines, still photographs, and yes, porno films. We fit ourselves behind the camera; in my case, I justified my voyeurism on the pages of a city tabloid. We were always watching. Only Mom with her canned performances in the living room came close to actually doing. Corny as Kansas and crazy as it was.

Then, we were all slightly torn around the edges, especially juxtaposed with Evan and Ellen who shared a typical habit of finishing each other's sentences. As when Ellen offered the reason they'd chosen their particular New Jersey suburb. "I want the kids to really know their grandparents," she said.

"And our office is just outside of Hoboken," Evan added, reaching for a cracker to catch the sliver of brie hanging from his knife.

A more normal couple I couldn't have invented. They were married. Had a house. A mortgage. Plans for children not yet born. It was everything I was supposed to want, yet imagining myself in their lives I felt restrained, as I'd been earlier when Mom gripped my biceps. Besieged by a string of wet sneezes, I longed to be on the set of an Alexis Calyx film.

I wiped my nose with a cocktail napkin and listened politely until we heard Aunt Lorraine's friend Kiki yell: "Gang way! Look out below!"

Everyone ran to the stairs. Aunt Lorraine sat at the top, strapped into the Baby Jane chair. She looked okay from where we stood, rather like a film director in the Yankee cap Kaminsky had given her and those tinted glasses. Yet, with her legs strapped at the calves and her bare feet poking out of her leggings, I thought if you tilted her on her back she would resemble the fallen turkey.

Aunt Lorraine pressed a button. "We have clearance, Houston," she said. "Geronimooooooooooh!"

"Ain't no stopping us now," Kiki said, and thus commenced the buzzing of the electronic conveyor belt. The rest of us stood quietly. Evan and Ellen looked captivated but alarmed, as if they were watching firemen burst into a burning building. My fears about the chair breaking down or catapulting Aunt Lorraine forward were assuaged by Kiki walking next to her. They'd been friends since before I was born, from their days of weekend trips to the Catskills, bingo tournaments, and bottomless glasses of bourbon and ginger ale. Kiki, whose proper name was Gertrude Sapperstein, lived around the corner, again since time immemorial, and worked in the meat department at the A&P.

"See, she loves it!" Hy said. "You love it!" Rowdy came running up with his video camera, and I thought his *Docudeath* would resemble something by Fellini or Almodovar. I laughed. Then I wanted to cry.

Meanwhile, Aunt Lorraine held tightly to her patent leather pocketbook. She reminded me of a toy figure. Nothing sinister like that damn Bermuda gun, but more like a fluffy gizmo out of a battery commercial: little old lady descending a staircase. I wanted to jump in her lap and ride down with her. If only I could be her pocketbook.

"How ya doing?" Rowdy asked.

"I feel like a piece of luggage going round and round."

At the bottom of the stairs, the chair screeched to a halt and, after a few awkward seconds, everyone cheered. I kneeled to help Kiki unfasten the safety belts. "Oy, I'm still hunched, you could mop the floor with my titties," Kiki said.

Aunt Lorraine laughed, her face so ruddy I might have forgotten she was sick but for the shiny head beneath her baseball cap and the bandages shrouded by her favorite sweatshirt, oversized and white, with swirls of gold and silver painted around a few strategically placed rhinestones. Casual with a flair, she always said of her style. A reaction to the many weekdays of dreary dresses worn to her bureaucratic job.

"Yo, yo, Aunt Lorraine, look here." Rowdy zoomed in on her face. "Tell us what you feel."

"Not so close, please." Aunt Lorraine flagged off the camera and rose from the chair. "I'm not one of Rachel's porno gals."

"You could have been in your day," I smiled, hoping Evan and Ellen had heard her say my name in conjunction with the word porno as they scooted around us and walked back into the living room. I wanted my outsider status confirmed for them.

"Porno? Like on cable?" Kiki said. We each locked onto one of Aunt Lorraine's arms and started the slow trek over the foyer and through the living room to the dining room table. "I get all the channels, Stevie hooked 'em up for nothing—now slow down, Lo, we're not running at Belmont. Rachey, you know my brother Stevie?"

"Of course she knows Stevie," Aunt Lorraine said. "He was at Louie's funeral."

"How do I know what she remembers?"

"Her father's funeral she should remember."

What I remember most about Dad's funeral was wishing Mom would come back from the hospital. Then, when she finally showed up, making her grand entrance with those nurses who looked like porn stars themselves, and fainting before the ceremony ended, I wished only that they would get her out of there before people started talking. I also remember feeling comforted that Aunt Lorraine was there with me.

At the step between the living room and dining room, Aunt Lorraine grabbed my wrist tightly. Kiki and I practically had to hoist her up, a feat that left me feeling sad and lonely, yet protective. I reminded myself that I would do anything she wanted.

We were settling Aunt Lorraine into her customary seat at the head of the table when Mom sauntered into the living room. Iridescent in her green lamé blouse and golden brown bouffant, she pivoted in front of Hy, stopping to give his cheek a kiss and then carefully wipe off the lipstick stain. "My god," Kiki said, "she looks like a lava lamp."

Mom beamed her way through the living room and headed over to us.

"Aren't you something," Aunt Lorraine said.

"Thank you, dear," Mom smiled, then turned to me. "I need you in the kitchen."

Inside, she said, "I wanted Hy and me on each end of the table, it's been a long time since we had a gentleman at the head of the table."

"A what?" I could barely speak. Aunt Lorraine had no hair, a hole from the catheter in her chest, and Mom was tormented over seating arrangements.

"You should have asked."

"Fine, go tell her to move."

"I can't do that."

"Well, don't look at me."

"All I'm saying is next time ask me." Mom opened the oven and started removing the casserole dishes. "Things are gonna be changing around here, you'll see."

"Yeah, she'll be dead." The words tasted like acid, but I didn't budge.

"That's not what I meant, you...ow! Goddinga, Hy!" Mom pulled her hand from the oven and started shaking it. The oven door bounced up with a bang.

"Are you okay?" I said.

"You see I'm not okay!" Mom shoved her index finger in between her lips and sucked it. Hy came running and, as if on cue, threw his arms around her.

"I burned my finger!"

"Here, let me see." Hy took my mother's hand and sat her down at the kitchen table. He patted her head, whispered in her ear as I stood awkwardly to the side.

"Don't just stand there, Rachel," Mom said. "We have to cut the turkey."

I was so angry I'd slipped into my statuesque mode, silent and glaring. Hy jumped up. "Man's work, Ray. I'll take care of it."

A wind of spices snared me as Hy opened the oven and leaned down before the steaming bird. I looked over and for a second saw the turkey's leg over Hy's ear, just as Tessa what's-her-name had enveloped Mark Vladimir with her thighs that day on the set. I was struck by a sudden need for Shade, and imagined myself crawling deep inside of her legs.

As it was, I stayed silent while Hy, following Mom's instructions, scooped the stuffing from the bird's stomach. It smelled of onions and oregano and had thick chunks of bread mixed with celery and giblets and juice. My stomach growled, and I felt as if I could devour the seventeen-pound bird and all of its complements myself. I hated that Mom's food could do this to me, that her turkey looked so damn delicious, its skin flecked with pepper and rosemary, and the occasional clove of garlic nestled against its torso.

Hy pulled back the turkey's skin with his fingertips and took a large fork and knife to it. "Gee, Mister, you sure know how to carve," Mom said, and they laughed together.

Pressure walled inside my face, behind my eyes. I wanted to rip the turkey to pieces with my bare hands and then pull the cloth from the dining room table so the china and crystal shattered, disrupting every sign of Thanksgiving Day propriety. Nothing had meaning. Nothing felt safe anymore...*Aunt Lorraine was really dying!*

I had to get out of the kitchen. Away from my mother and her turkey-carving man. I brought the bread baskets into the dining room and took yoga breaths along the way to cap the sadness, the anger, the hatred. Mom and I avoided each other's eyes as we passed between the kitchen and dining room. Soon the food was out and everyone took their seats. Hy ended up sitting to the left of Mom, and next to me, and Aunt Lorraine looked happy at the head of the table with Kiki on one side of her and Rowdy on the other.

We ate quickly and quietly, as was our habit. Away from the family, I had to check myself so I wouldn't finish first, but here there was always someone with greasy fingers beating me to the serving spoon for seconds. Usually it was Rowdy, who stacked his plate so high he barely had room to cut his meat. He was a lefty, too. Poor Ellen kept bumping up against his wandering elbow as Aunt Lorraine asked her the story of her life this time.

Rowdy reached into the turkey platter, pitching his fork in one piece after another, looking dismayed.

"What is the matter with you?" Mom asked him.

"There's no ass," he said. "How can you have no ass?"

"I see an ass," Kiki stared at him.

"I got it this year," Aunt Lorraine smiled.

"Oh man," Rowdy said. "That's my favorite part."

"Just like your father," Kiki said. "Louie used to love the ass. And turtles, too. Remember that guy who sold the turtles out of a plastic bag? Only Louie would eat them."

"Down in Bermuda, we ate little hens," Mom said. Her face, like the rest of ours, was red from food and wine. We were so pink, so precious; skin so thin you could see the blood running through our veins. "Hy, tell them about the hens."

"It was unreal." Hy shoveled a fork full of string beans into his mouth. "You'da thought they were pigeons or something."

"The chinks eat pigeons," Rowdy said.

"They do not," Hy said. "Who told you that?"

"Nobody, it's one of those things everyone knows."

"Hy, tell them about the hotel," Mom said.

"Hotel shmotel," Kiki said. "I want to hear more about your porno, Rachey." I almost spit up the water in my mouth. But the look of horror on Mom's face made it all worthwhile. Her saying we didn't need to hear about *that* only sealed my victory.

Kiki went on talking. "We went to a strip place in Texas, for my niece's bachelorette. It was a riot, all those boys with their dickies packed in little pouches, how do they get them in there? I put a few dollars in the elastic, my niece and her friends were saying, 'Aunt Gertie, you're crazy.'"

"Our room was right on the beach," Mom interjected. "At night you could see all the stars, the big dipper and everything. Right Hy?"

Aunt Lorraine touched Kiki's arm. "You should see the movies she got," she said.

"Yeah, what channel? I got free cable, all the channels."

"We walked in the moonlight, didn't we?" Mom shoved Hy's arm, but he seemed taken with the conversation at our end of the table, where Aunt Lorraine was explaining to Kiki that she would not find these movies on cable. She would have to get them from the video store or from me, because I had friends in the business.

"Like that famous boy, what's his name again?"

"You mean Robbie Rod?" I said.

"That's the one," Aunt Lorraine smiled. "And talk about hanging. He's got the biggest ever, isn't that so hun?"

"Well technically, no. They say he's twelve inches, but rumor has it he was never really that big, and anyway some guys are thirteen, fourteen inches...really big." I felt naughty discussing penis size over the din of forks clashing with plates and water glasses being refilled, especially when I could tell from Mom's face how badly I was behaving. Quite frankly, it inspired me.

"Twelve inches sounds pretty big to me, that's like a ruler," Kiki said.

"It is a ruler," I said. "But the thing about Robbie Rod wasn't just his size, he knew how to use it."

"Is this the same Robbie Rod of the *Pleasure Squad* fame?" Evan smiled.

"The one and only," I said. It had been the *Pleasure Squad* series that made RR famous. He played a detective.

Ellen grimaced at her husband, as if he'd just said his pants were on fire. "What?" he said. "It was years ago, I was just a kid."

"Rachel knows him," Aunt Lorraine said proudly.

"Well, we've met a few times." My mind drifted back to the set, how RR had been breeding bad karma, because he'd backed out of the production after his fight with Claire Blue but hung around barking orders at the other actors. His money was still tied up in the movie, he argued. Alexis humored him; I started feeling sorry for him. It isn't easy watching your career slip away. Once, just after a marathon conversation with Shade, I even fantasized taking him up on his offer to fly off to Las Vegas with him for Thanksgiving. Apparently, he had a house there.

"So what's he like?" Evan asked.

"Actually, he's just a regular guy," I said.

And the questions kept coming. It was similar to the way I'd felt in that restaurant with RR and Alexis, as if the company I kept, this job I'd taken, made me more libertine than most. A sexual revolutionary by default. It didn't matter that I was all talk, that I needed Silver Ray to help me along. I knew my coup was complete when Mom threw her napkin on her plate and took it into the kitchen. Hy followed her. The rest of us started stacking our plates and passing them around the table.

"I heard those guys aren't allowed to have sex for weeks before a shoot," Evan said.

"Evan!" Ellen looked at him, half-smiling, as she lifted a stack of plates to bring into the kitchen. She kidded him about any more secrets she should know before she got pregnant, and he made a crack about wearing women's underwear and everyone laughed but me. I felt newly kindred with those of aberrant desire.

"All those porno guys got implants anyway," Rowdy said.

"No, you putz," Kiki said. "They use pumps. Harry used to have one, like a bicycle pump. Push, push, push, and your weenie blows up. You know those, Rachey?"

"No, but some men eat raw onions." I said this quite pleased with my expertise, though I knew it was probably a Mark Vladimir quirk and not a trend.

"Onions?" Kiki said.

"Cross my heart, I saw it myself."

"Blech!" Kiki said. "All this talk and I forgot I gotta pee." She left the table just as Hy returned.

Ellen helped Mom transport the dirty dishes and platters into the kitchen, making me feel guilty for sitting. The women always cleared, while the men sat smoking cigarettes with their belts unbuckled. But Mom had banned cigarettes from the house, so Rowdy went outside to smoke, leaving me at the table with Hy, Evan, and Aunt Lorraine, whose sickness had given her a gender dispensation of sorts. But I felt that way, too. Different from the rest of them. A woman who travels to porn sets. A woman who masturbates. A woman who kisses other women.

I could hear the coffee pot gurgling in the kitchen as I talked to Evan. Like many people I found myself talking to in New York, he confessed that he'd always wanted to be a writer himself; someday he would take off a few months and write that book he had in him. I said someday I would find a family business to go into. Rowdy ambled in with his video camera. Kiki followed him shaking sprinkles of water from her fingers. Ellen and Mom brought out dessert: a pecan pie, Hy's favorite, a marble pound cake, fruit salad, and an assortment of colorful cookies from the bakery. Watching my mother walk in and out, conducting the rest of them with her burned index finger now covered in gauze, I felt guilty and wanted to make up with her. "Everything looks great," I said. But she ignored me.

"Yeah, doesn't it?" Hy said. He picked up his coffee cup. "A toast to my beautiful Stella. What a meal, doll. What a day!"

We all went to sip from our coffee cups, but Mom stopped us. "What? Why'd you stop?" she said. "Tell them the rest."

"No, Stella, I told you not yet."

"I'm tired of waiting, they're gonna find out sooner or later."

"It's not the right time, Stella."

"What?" Evan turned from Hy to Mom. "What's going on?"

"We're engaged, we're getting married next fall!"

"Hey congrats, man!" Rowdy put down his camera and started clapping his hands. When nobody joined in, he stopped.

"You're what?" Ellen said.

"We're getting married," Mom said.

"I can't believe this," Evan said. "You hardly know each other."

"I wanted to tell you, but—"

"Mom hasn't been dead six months!"

"Six months?" I said and felt Kiki kick me underneath the table. Hy had been coming around for at least a year, and this was the first we'd heard about his wife. We all assumed she was long dead.

"Wait a minute, you were seeing her when...with Mom...." Evan's voice shook. Hy buried his head in his hands. Evan stared at him for a second, then put down his coffee cup and bolted from the table. Ellen stood up to follow him, but Hy grabbed her arm. "Come on, Ellie? You gotta understand," he pleaded. The sacks beneath his eyes sunk lower and lower. Ellen shook him off and ran out the front door with Rowdy trailing after her with his video camera.

"Let them go, Hy," Mom said.

"Oh, babydoll, why?" Hy whined, reduced to shambles. I thought he might cry and, at that moment, saw he was everything Dad wasn't. My father would have beaten the crap out of his son before letting him run away from the dinner table. Then he would have called Mom names as their screaming began, a match of twitching jugular veins and flicking wrists, pink blotches on white skin.

Not Hy, he called her babydoll and stroked her arm. I felt sorry for him, caught between her and his family, but weighing the facts as I knew them, my sympathy had its limits. Even Dad, I believe, wouldn't have cheated on his dying wife.

"I'll be right back," Hy said softly and went to catch his family. The rest of us were silent; Kiki, Aunt Lorraine, and I huddled on one side of the table, Mom on the other.

"Stop it! Stop staring at me!" Mom slammed her chair into the table and rose defiantly as if she herself hadn't smashed the evening to pieces.

"Nobody's staring," I said, afraid she might faint, or at least try it, but she'd already sent people running from the table. Fainting would be redundant.

"Six months!" She imitated me, her nose scrunched up and eyes glaring. "You just can't let me have any happiness, can you? All of you. Jealous bitches!"

She walked off screaming Hy's name until the front door slammed behind her.

"She is totally nuts," I said.

"No, just sad," Aunt Lorraine nodded. "She could have had some life, but nothing was ever enough, just like your father. They were too much alike."

"Louie was lucky," Kiki said. "He saw it coming and got out."

"You're giving him too much credit," I said, thinking of all the times Dad had come from work smelling like scotch, how the union local had called that day. *Louie's in the hospital, a metal beam whacked him in the kisser.* If they knew he was drunk, they didn't say anything, allowing him and, later, Mom to collect disability.

"He had a good heart, until it stopped working," Aunt Lorraine said. She smiled beneath her Yankee cap, and though her rheumy eyes were trimmed with yellow spots and broken blood vessels, she seemed more alive than ever. I remembered how she and Dad had always clung to each other, how they sat together so many evenings listening to the saddest music I'd ever heard, tango music. Songs about love and longing and war. Songs that made my father cry. Aunt Lorraine was the only one who understood his tears, the only one he never hit or berated. Aside from me.

"Mind you, I'm not making any excuses," she said. "People pay for their lives."

"Not in Brooklyn, they don't," Kiki said. She stuck her fork in the middle of the pecan pie and shoved a huge chunk in her mouth.

Aunt Lorraine and I dipped our forks into the dish. I shook the can of whipped cream but stopped at the sudden flash on Aunt Lorraine's face. She wasn't supposed to have any sugar.

"What are you waiting for?" she said. We shared a quick second of recognition: yes, honey, we both know what's going on, and I still want the whipped cream. All of my life I feared doing the wrong thing. I was terrified of, say, not following doctors orders or not clearing my credit card balance the day I received the bill. But I had been to the porn set and back, I'd made a pass at Shade the other night, I wasn't even reading newspapers anymore, and the world went on just the same.

So I shot a stream of whipped cream on each of our forks and then built a sculpture like the Colosseum in the middle of the pie. The three of us sat swallowing whipped cream and laughing, and I was happy in the sick sweetness, happy until I spotted Rowdy standing against the wall, his spindly fingers hugging the video camera to his chest, with his shoulders jerking and tears streaming down his cheeks.

Bang, Bang, You're...

First the shot went off. One long echoed bang, as if a fleet of trucks had backfired simultaneously. My ears rang, dazed as eyes navigating the aftermath of a photographer's flash. Then I heard the man scream.

Heads ducked down; fear crept up my back. People dropped their signs, rushing back and forth in every direction like a scene from an old Japanese monster movie.

Shade squeezed my arm. "You okay?"

I took a deep breath, and my lips shook. "Yeah, you?"

She nodded, clasped her hand tightly around mine, and together we elbowed our way out of the police barricades, which the union leaders had decorated with colorful Christmas lights. We spotted Tony standing by the coffee shop. Shade let go of my hand, and I wished we were back in the crowd, our fingers locked as we bounced like electrons between the bodies of strangers.

We joined Tony and asked him what happened.

"Some idiot machinist was packing a forty-five and the thing went off. Got'im in the foot."

"His own foot?" Shade said.

"He was carrying a gun?"

"Yes, he shot himself, and yes, he had a gun. That's kind of a no-brainer." He reached into his pocket, pulled out a pouch of tobacco, and started rolling a cigarette.

"A gun! What was he doing with a gun?" I had to scream above the bedlam. The horns and megaphones. People shouting. The ominous wailing of police cars and an emergency rescue van.

A few reporters mingled amid the crowd scribbling on pads and flicking their cell phones. The three of us noticed them simultaneously. Shade zipped up her olive green leather jacket and turned her back to them. Bloated clouds wrestled with the wind above. Tony kicked the ground and leaned back against a parked car, almost too casually. I wondered if he'd heard my question about the gun. He bit a string of tobacco from the end of his cigarette and spit it into the gutter. "I can't even afford real cigarettes."

"You never could," Shade said.

"No, I used to be able to, I just didn't want to. There's a big difference." He exhaled, looking defeated, angry, as if pushed the wrong way he might explode. A lot of people out here looked that way. Striker's pose.

"Are you still editing?" Shade asked Tony, and again I couldn't believe they weren't talking about the shooting. As if it were innocuous, like the crack of my toy gun from Bermuda.

"Yeah, I had a couple of days at *EgoEast* this week. Magazines are so funny. Nobody works. They all come in at ten, dressed like models. Then they go to lunch."

"Wait a minute, what's going on here?" I interjected. "Am I hallucinating or did some guy just shoot himself?"

They both laughed, looked at me as if I were a kid asking where babies come from. I felt like an idiot. "Where have you been, Rachel?" Tony dropped his cigarette and crushed it with his dirty sneakers.

Shade and I crossed stares. She winked at me, as if to say my secret was safe with her. I wondered which secret we were protecting: the job, the porno, our kiss. "She's been hiding out in Brooklyn."

"You don't have TV there?" Tony said. "They've been tipping delivery trucks and dumping papers in the Hudson like crazy. The other night they pummeled a driver so badly he wound up in the hospital."

"It kicked off every channel," Shade added.

"Really, look," Tony said. He shoved his neck to the left, where a few union leaders were surrounded by microphones, cameras, and tape recorders. Nobody had told me any of this when I'd been here last week. Then again, I'd basically signed in and left unnoticed.

Today, having a few free hours and wanting to glom on to their union solidarity, I followed Shade and Tony to The Corral, where I heard more gruesome tales of the line. Apparently, strikers were now spitting paint through plastic straws at anyone who crossed, marking their treachery in chicken-shit yellow. Then there were the scab-beatings and midnight truck raids. Tony said he'd gone along one night. He was so drunk he couldn't get the stocking over his head and ended up passing out in the back seat of a car belonging to a bundler or pressman, he couldn't remember. Sunrise found him in the car alone as the rest of the insurgents celebrated over breakfast.

I should have been appalled by the violence, moved perhaps to action or indignation, but hard as I tried, I couldn't bring myself to care. All I wanted was for Tony to leave so I could be alone with Shade.

This happened sooner than expected, as the strike had been a boon to Tony's popularity. He strutted between tables as if he were at a wedding where he knew just about everyone in the room. Shade also received her share of nods, and I had to work hard to keep down my jealousy.

"Are you drinking these days?" she asked after Tony left.

"Sure, why not?" I had nothing to do until Ethan's Christmas party later. I was bringing Robbie Rod, whom I'd ended up inviting the day before. He was saying he liked the way I watched people and the way I listened, intently, with my entire body. "Most people hate keeping secrets," I replied. "They'll tell you anything if you look at them right."

"You want to divulge a few secrets, Silver? I promise I'll watch."

He had stared as if he already knew every one of my secrets. I blushed, but managed to allay the tension. "I have no secrets, RR," I said.

"Good. Me neither."

"Good."

"So let's have dinner tomorrow."

"Actually, I've got another idea," I said, and before I knew it he'd agreed to come with me to Ethan's party, and I immediately thought, what have I done? How can I get out of this? Although I smiled at RR and laughed about the fun we'd have, I feared the wrath of Alexis, who certainly wouldn't approve of me dating her ex-husband, feared the reception of my pedigreed colleagues, feared the thought of meeting him for drinks before the party. It all seemed too intimate.

Neither had I found the right moment to tell any of this to Shade, who'd put in our order for a pitcher of kamikazes. "The preferred cocktail of striking reporters," she assured me, adopting the Scarlett O'Hara voice she affected in bars.

"Since when?"

She shifted her head back and forth a few times then sighed. "Okay, look, I'm sick of tequila. Tequila makes me batty, and it's all anybody drinks around here. That and watered down beer. I feel like I'm back in college. Besides, we need a new ritual. We *need* kamikazes, okay?"

"Okay."

We smiled until it embarrassed me. I looked around the bar, dark and smoky with wooden chairs and brown formica tables. It could have been any bar, in any city, anywhere. I did recognize a few people, and I caught the scent of nostalgia in the air. It would be a stretch to say I missed these people whose names I could barely keep straight, but acquaintances made the world whole, gave it context. Since the strike my professional context had changed, at the very least it wore less clothing.

"I don't know, Slivowitz," Shade sighed, and I thought she might be tired of me, frustrated by our situation. Her every word or gesture, no matter how innocuous, seemed coded. A sentence, a smile, a tap on the wrist, nothing was what it was. I felt as if I were studying a foreign language, unsure of my translations and afraid to speak. You might call it social aphasia. Or performance anxiety.

Salvation came in a silver cauldron. Shade filled two shot glasses with the pale, lemony liquid and handed me one. "Here's to never being boring," she said. We clicked our glasses together and drank.

The sourball elixir chafed my throat, and I feared throwing up. Shade refilled our glasses. "Again," she said. "And none of your one-for-me-one-for-the-floor routine."

"You knew?"

"I'm omniscient."

"Then why are you trying to get me drunk?"

"I don't know, you think it'll work?"

I tipped back my shot glass, drank the contents, and slammed the glass down on the bar. "Yes," I said and laughed.

"Slivowitz." She pivoted toward me, propping her head up with a bent elbow. "There's something I have to tell you." The look in her eye finished the sentence...*and you're not going to like it.* Tina Macadam, I thought, feeling the blood drain slowly from my face.

"I'm going home for a few weeks, at least through the holidays."

"That's it?"

She shrugged.

"You're such an alarmist, why do you do that? I thought it was something bad."

"Well it is sort of, I'm leaving tomorrow." Her brow crinkled, her mustard eyes clouding like the late afternoon sky. Then again, I was looking through a kamikaze-colored lens. She refilled our glasses. "So I was thinking we should do something tonight."

"Oh god." I buried my head in my hands, feeling guilty. In my mind I saw myself calling RR and canceling. Ethan wouldn't know the difference.

"What?" Shade touched my shoulder, again asking what, and I felt as if I'd cheated on her, which was ridiculous when she was the one who kept pulling away. Guilt slowly gave way to resentment and I thought: why should I change my plans just because she's leaving town tomorrow?

"Look, if you can't just say so," she said.

"No, it's not that, I mean that's part of it, but..."

"I can't hear you." She pushed my shoulder back so I had to lift my head up. We stared. I reached for the kamikaze Shade had poured and drank it in one quick gulp.

"I'm going to Ethan's Christmas party, and I invited Robbie Rod. There, now you own it with me."

"You're going out with that porn star?"

"He's an entrepreneur, he only used to be a porn star."

"I don't care what he is, I don't give a shit about him," she said, raising her voice just enough to make me wary. "How can you do this to me?"

"To you? So I'm supposed to be exclusive in this unrequited thing."

"You still don't get it!" A few people turned to look at us; the bartender lowered his eyes in our direction.

"Well, then start explaining." I reached into my pocket and pulled out a twenty dollar bill. "Because you know what? I'm really sick of hearing how you know everything and I know nothing, just because I've never been with another woman."

"Put your money back," Shade said, but I stuck the bill on the bar.

"I want to go."

"Why?"

"Because we can't talk here."

"What are you afraid of, you big traitor? You scab!"

"Don't call me that!" More heads turned toward us, their half-familiar faces slapping me with sobriety. "Are you crazy? You want to get me splattered!"

Shade bit her lip, then turned her head away. I stood, swung my bag over my shoulder, and leaned in close. "If you want to talk I'll be outside."

I walked out into a bullet-gray sky, nervous that Shade hadn't followed me. As much as I wanted to run back and throw my arms around her, I had to admit it felt sort of cool being the one who walked off. *Cool.* Another word waxed in multiplicity and overrated: if being cool was so great, why was I left tipsy and alone with the wind slapping the collar of my pea coat up against my face?

Craving a cigarette, I bummed one from a young woman in nylon sweats with a walkman attached to her ears. I saddled up against a car in the lot next to The Corral. To my right was the coffee shop, in front of me was the picket line where the remaining strikers huddled together, occasionally flouting a poster or screaming an obscenity in the winds full of flying trash. She should have come after me already.

I watched a man duck around the coffee shop. He moved nervously, looking back and forth at the strikers as he walked toward me. His coat was similar to mine but for a few streaks of bright yellow paint: a scab. The first I could actually identify. It made me think of the yellow star the Nazis had stamped on my grandfather, marking him for death. Despite the Italian flag patches on my jeans, the visits to the priest, the name change, I couldn't shake his jaundiced yellow from my sleeve.

When I was in my early teens, I used to dream the Nazis came to Brooklyn. They took up residence at the local synagogue and began their systematic genocide. Bay Ridge started looking like East Germany before the wall came down. Through the burnt-out buildings and fallen bricks, I wandered, a massive, gold Italian horn swinging over my flat chest. My job was to find Jews in hiding and turn them in. I gave up my entire family, but that wasn't enough. What saved me, finally, was sucking Hitler's cock, because everyone knows Jewish girls didn't do that. I had survived, but I was alone—a closeted Jew in the new and improved, ethnically cleansed Bay Ridge. The biggest traitor of them all.

As the scab came closer, our eyes met in a passing stare. He must have guessed I was the enemy, although he had no clue I didn't give a shit about the fight. He couldn't have known I was more likely to drop to my knees in sympathy than to spit paint or tip a truck. Maybe Shade was right, I was more scab than striker.

Above me the sky rumbled, a raindrop tickled my nose. I tossed my cigarette and through the charcoal air traced its arc to the ground.

"Good, you're still here," Shade said. I looked up and found her standing a few feet in front of me. Her hair was pulled back tightly against her head, and her eyes looked swollen. "I'm really sorry," she said.

"Maybe the kamikazes weren't such a good idea."

"No, it's not that. It's like all of a sudden everything went red."

"That's what serial killers say." I pulled my collar up against my chin and smiled at her. Around us, the mist and drizzle felt like anticipation. We were still for a while, not saying anything, just staring. I swear her eyes said take me home. "Look, I can cancel tonight," I said. "I was going to say that before you freaked out."

"Don't do that. Maybe we need some time."

A crack of thunder and the raindrops got hard. In the distance I could see strikers sprinting to the coffee shop as Shade and I battled the rain amid the flashing lights of The Corral, and I wished we were at a cheap motel in a place neither one of us knew.

She wiped a raindrop from her nose, sniffled. Her hand flung up to hail a cab, and one screeched to a halt in front of us. "You want it?" she said.

"You take it." I held the door open as she climbed inside. Before shutting the door, I bent down into the stuffy heat and asked her if she wanted to come with us tonight.

"Get in with the competition, are you crazy?"

"Competition? Is that what's going on?"

"You tell me, later," she smiled. "Now, get out of the rain, Slivowitz. You're all wet."

At that she pulled the door shut. The cab took off, cutting a yellow trail through the pouring rain. Had I not been too chicken-shit yellow myself, I would have jumped in with her. Silver Ray might have. Rachel Silver stopped at the Korean deli on the corner and bought a pack of cigarettes before going home.

"I didn't know you smoked," RR said. We'd just finished an awkward cocktail hour, during which I chugged a couple of Cokes and stammered into a monologue about the man who shot himself on the picket line. RR said little. But he did notice I'd gotten a haircut since I'd last seen him. So had he. He didn't like his cut, said it was a drag he could no longer make a ponytail. Mine was a different story. He told me he liked the way I let it dry naturally instead of straightening it with a blow dryer. He said I looked vibrant, less professional.

"I don't usually buy cigarettes," I said, tossing the used match and inhaling deeply as we pushed through the cold, black night. Veins of highway crisscrossed on Canal Street. We headed south toward the industrial theme park, where Ethan and others in the media gentry had in the past couple of decades settled. It was said to be very chic, but the vacant streets and loft buildings looked lonely in the dark.

Again, uncomfortable with RR's silence, I tried to push the cigarette conversation. "I hated people like me when I really smoked."

He said nothing.

"You know the type, always bumming, never buying."

Still not a word. I smoked seriously, as if the act itself were an art. "I always said no way would I ever be that kind of tiresome grub, but..."

"We all become what we hate sooner or later. It's called growing up."

I nodded, because I couldn't think of a response. RR had a way of stating things so simply they curtailed further conversation, his words resonating, the gaps and long pauses only making them seem more profound. Warhol again. The school of silent geniuses. Perhaps I'd spent too much time around journalists, but most people I knew used words and sentences to project a bit of themselves onto others. Listen closely to most conversations and you'll find little more than dueling soliloquies. RR wasn't like that. From what I could tell he used language to get back to silence.

I decided he must be the kind of guy people thought of when they spoke about the strong, silent type. Although I usually liked more talkative men, it was nice not to battle for conversation time. We could take in the scenery, enjoy the night. But soon the streaming cars and the click of my heels against the concrete grew ominous. The air felt thicker, as if someone had sabotaged the climate control out there on the cold, damp street, and left me in the suffocating silence wishing he would say something. Anything at all.

Resisting another monologue of my own, I concentrated on walking. The same platform boots that had served me well inside my apartment were a risk on these cracked sidewalks, still slick from the evening's rain. That I managed to make it the few blocks to Ethan's without falling was remarkable. My sacrifice in comfort proved worthwhile when we stepped inside Ethan's loft and, upon relinquishing our coats to a man in a tuxedo, I peeped at myself in the mirrored foyer and thought I looked good, a bit like Alexis with my boots, tight black cocktail dress, and newly tousled curls flowing down my back. I even had her ex-husband along for the ride. As we followed the trail of black and white balloons into the huge living area, I noticed people, particularly those who knew me, doing a double take as if they'd made a mistake and blinking might correct the image. It was him, too. The man was ridiculous, with his fashionably spiked hair more brown and less gray than I remembered, and those tight black trousers. He looked like a rock star middleaging from pop icon to serious artist.

I couldn't believe my own moxie, bringing a famous porn star to a party full of journalists, the subgroup of my acquaintance from that fancy journalism school I'd slipped into on my virginity and a dream. I'd always felt the fraud in those ivy-covered buildings, but showed them all when I landed a job right out of school at the daily in Jersey and within a year tripled my circulation in the move to Miami. I finally hit the top when the *News* came calling and returned to New York where I promptly lost my job. Showed them all, didn't I?

We walked to the bar where RR ordered a Coke for me and a beer for himself. Making our way toward the windows with the Hudson River view, I heard Ethan call my name. He was smack in the middle of the blue-chip crowd. We joined them, and Ethan eyed RR as I'd hoped he would. He might have had a pregnant wife, but I had a bona fide boy-toy.

I said hello and introduced my friend, Robbie…

"Rob Vaughn." RR shook hands with Ethan and smiled at everyone else. I quick-referenced people to their jobs for him: Joan Pinchett and Harry Lansing from *Wall Street Week*, Susan from the computer magazine, Anne from the morning radio show, Jason with his theater magazine and blond boyfriend George, an actor. As I spoke, RR's name haunted me like a record sample…*Rob Vaughn…Rob Vaughn…Rob Vaughn. His last name was Vaughn?* It sounded familiar, like somebody else's name. Later, I would remember that it actually was somebody else's name, another actor, from straight films and television, but right then, in Ethan's living room, I was simply shocked that he had a last name other than "Rod" and that I didn't know it. I'd never thought to ask. Amazing, what gets by when you stop asking questions.

I was the journalist without questions, and RR my accomplice for the evening. He took the attention away from my downward mobility, although I started getting nervous when Ethan asked him where he worked.

"Mostly in Vegas," RR said.

"No," Ethan said. "I meant what do you do?"

"Little of this, little of that."

"He's got his own business, in film," I added, afraid of what else RR might reveal and also to keep up the mystery. Upon hearing the word film the little networkers smiled. Cartoon bubbles springing from their heads might have said: Synergy. The conversation then turned to questions about the strike, although I wasn't confident I could answer them being away from the picket line as much as I was.

"It must be terrible," Anne said.

"Yeah, I—" I started to speak, but the circle overwhelmed me, a chorus of concerned eyes and tisk-tisks. I couldn't follow who was saying what:

"It can't last forever."

"I only wish I had a few weeks with nothing to do."

"At least you can freelance."

"I'm actually—"

"Has anyone heard from Peter?"

"Still in China."

And that was that. Too much talk of suffering made people nervous. They wanted just enough to empathize and think better her than me. Only Joan Pinchett, the bitch, kept staring at us. It figured. She'd been my nemesis back at Columbia, always showing up at the same events as I did and trying to listen in on my conversations in the telephone room; she'd even chosen a similar thesis topic on community policing. I knew I'd finally beaten her when RR offered to get her a drink, and she said "No!" as if she'd seen a roach crawling between the miniature quiches.

"What's her problem?" RR said.

"I think she recognized you, but she'd never admit it. She's a Republican."

"So am I."

"Get out!"

He rolled his eyes, shrugged. "I don't like people screwing with my money."

"I should have known."

"Another Coke?"

"No, something stronger, something Republican."

"Scotch?"

"Champagne," I said. "But only if it's really expensive."

He laughed, one eyebrow crept up his forehead, and I knew I'd scored points for amusing him. "Don't go anywhere," he said. I traced his shoulders as he disappeared into the crowd, leaving me by myself. I thought about barging back into the group now a few feet away, but how? Cocktail parties had never been my forte. Better to pretend I was happy alone, enjoying the three-piece jazz band. Better to turn and look out the window. It was a foggy night. I could barely make out the Jersey skyline, and the Verrazano was a mesh of string and clouds, as if someone had taken a thumb and tried to smudge out the passage to Bay Ridge, disconnecting Brooklyn from the rest of the country and taking Aunt Lorraine away from me. I wondered if she was playing backgammon with Rowdy or watching an Alexis Calyx movie. What a strange bond for us to share, though I did take comfort in it.

A man came up behind me and by his smell, a woody scent that reminded me of my father, I knew who it was before turning around.

"Your friend's no regular studio honcho, is he?" Ethan said.

"You are a perceptive fellow."

"Go on, where'd you pick him up?" His voice was rushed, as if he had to know who my date was before he could move forward with his evening. I smiled and looked off into the party. The trio played an instrumental version of "The Lady is a Tramp," heavy on the tenor sax. A song about a woman who might buy a man for pleasure.

"Well?" Ethan said.

"It's embarrassing but...I used an escort service."

"Oh please, you're too frigid to pay for it."

"Maybe I have to pay for it to get what I want."

Ethan dropped his jaw, grunted, and eyed me curiously. As if he were running a computer check to see if my name cross-referenced with escort service. Before he could say anything, Jason and George broke in between us. "I hope we're interrupting something," Jason said.

"Not at all," Ethan said.

"Tell them the truth," I said, then turned to George and Jason. "He's mad I brought a gigolo to his party."

"A gigolo?" Ethan said. "What agency did you get him from?"

"Boys-R-Us," I said.

"Good on you, ducky," Jason said.

"You believe that crap?" Ethan huffed and shook his head back and forth before excusing himself.

Jason and George smiled at each other. "Boys-R-Us," Jason said.

"Uh-huh."

"It must be quite exclusive with that kind of personnel."

"What do you mean?"

"Really, sugar, we could spot a star such as your friend in a churchyard," George said in the Mississippi drawl that always made his words sound slightly lascivious. "There is no way you could afford that boy, not on strike."

I laughed out loud; they knew too much. "Please, don't tell Ethan."

"Fess up," George said. "Where'd you meet the movie star?"

So I told them how I'd come to arrive at the party with Robbie Republican on my arm, although I was wary of too many people knowing about my ghostwriting job. Having work, I often felt as guilty as a splattered scab, especially after the frustration and chaos I'd witnessed today. But I had to admit I liked the image my new job conferred. As if I had an inside line to the mystical forces of sexuality. My date a tenured member of the sexual cognoscenti, it followed that I was wild and exciting in bed. Need I state the power this syllogism—fallacious though it may have been—might work upon a woman who'd entered her thirties convinced she was a lousy lay? It was as if in my Silver Ray mind I'd become multiply orgasmic. And the image was contagious. Even Jason and George seemed more impressed than they would have been had I simply rented RR through Boys-R-Us.

Turns out, my old friends were porn aficionados, confessing to me and RR who'd just returned with my ritzy champagne that they had a closet full of movies, which was no surprise, although I was confounded by their footnote: most of the collection was heterosexual hard-core. "I don't get it," I said to Jason. "You haven't been within ten feet of a vagina since you were born, but you're into watching girls."

"Oh, no, that's not it at all," Jason said. "When I watch, I am the woman. You don't realize, but this man you're with," he turned to RR, "I mean, begging your pardon, Mr. Vaughn."

"Go for it," RR said, and I wondered if Jason had known RR's last name before he'd said it earlier. The word slid from his lips so easily.

"This man," Jason said, pushing his fingertips against his chest for emphasis, "he's every bottom's fantasy."

RR burst out laughing. "I love gay guys."

"Not as much as we love you, dear."

They all laughed. I didn't really understand what was going on, but thought better of saying anything. Instead, I looked around and noticed the loft had emptied considerably. I was nervous about what to do next, whether I would go home with Mr. Rob Vaughn and whether thinking this made me a bottom.

Jason, too, remarked on the thinning crowd and said they should be going. They had to catch Tricky's drag act in the West Village and invited us to come along. "Tricky would just die to meet a celebrity like yourself," George smiled.

He had no trouble convincing me, and RR said he was ready to leave as soon as we'd arrived, though I never would have known, he seemed so comfortable. On the way out Harry Lansing pulled RR and me aside. "See I've got this thing, this script," he said. "Well, it's not actually finished, it's more in the conceptional stage, but it's dynamite. In fact it's so great I'm hesitant to tell you. You are in the business, that's what she said, right?"

RR nodded, confirming my stretch of the word film earlier. Although he could have been a big-time movie producer listening to Harry Lansing give up his precious idea as if he'd been fed truth serum. His movie was a thriller about an ambitious young stock broker who discovers that aliens have taken over the Bloomberg numbers on his computer. "But these aliens don't look like any aliens we've ever seen before," said Harry. "They're tiny and they live in colonies, like ant colonies, and that's how they do it. How they get into the computer system. It's kind of like *Wall Street* meets *Independence Day.*"

"It sounds more like a hacker movie," RR said.

"How do you figure?"

"Aliens and computers."

"Talk about a post-millennial bug," I said.

"No," Harry said. "I really want it to be a moral story, about the broker. All stories are about people. We know this, right Rachel? Anyway, see, this broker's got the aliens feeding him insider information, so in the end he's got to choose between making money and saving himself. In the process, of course, he also saves the world."

"Of course," I said.

RR removed a card from his wallet and handed it to Harry. "Call me at my office," he said and then turned to me. "You ready?"

A few feet away I asked, "Was that your real card?"

"Yeah."

"Why'd you give it to him? He's going to be calling you every day."

"It's a good idea." He led me toward the foyer where we retrieved our coats.

"So?"

RR held out my coat for me. "I know people, I can do things," he said, and I wondered whether his words were meant to humor me or if before my very eyes he was becoming the person I'd invented. Either way I giggled as I turned and slipped my hands through the armholes of my coat, then felt his hand linger on my left shoulder, a soft touch that seemed characteristic of a famous director or Hollywood moneyman. Rob Vaughn. The guy who knows people.

Snug in my coat, I pivoted to face him. He was smiling seductively, like something I'd seen in *Sensurround.* "You don't believe a word I say, do you Silver?" he said, and I knew then that he would never be anything but RR to me.

Mirroring his flirtation, I said, "I thought you made porn films."

"No, I make money."

"And you really liked his idea?"

His eyeballs slid sideways, then back to me. "No."

We both burst out laughing.

"I like your laugh." He led me away from the coat check. "It's healthy, much lighter than the rest of you."

"Thanks," I said. "I think."

We arrived at the front door where we met the boys and said goodbye to a surly Ethan standing with his arm around Fran, who according to Jason and George was a total LGQ. "Low Glamour Quotient," Jason whispered to me on the way downstairs, making me self-conscious about my own glamour quotient.

"Give her a break, she's pregnant."

"Oh, please. The only reason Ethan married her is for her trust fund. Everybody knows that boy still has his face up every tunnel south of Ninety-sixth Street. I don't think he ever really got over you."

"Then he's a fool," I said, though I felt foolish myself. Two months ago I'd been one of Ethan's tunnels. The night he told me Fran was pregnant and slammed into me, brutally, as if I were the one usurping his freedom. Me, the quintessential bridge-and-tunnel gal. They come in, park, party, and then return to the clean streets of the suburbs. I tried to imagine it being any different with a porn star. Or with a woman. It suddenly seemed possible.

Down in the street the wind coiled around us, blowing my hair in a thousand different directions. "I always thought you were too good for him," Jason said. "You're a total dish."

Sweet of him, but I felt like Medusa. I hoped my nose wasn't greasy and the pink lipstick hadn't lodged in the runnels of my lips, pursed as they were in disbelief. Jason smiled. "Really, as far as HGQs go, you're off the scale. Thank you, Robert," he raised his eyebrows provocatively at RR who held open the back door of a cab for us. At that moment I did feel charmed, though in a Cinderella kind of way, as if I were on borrowed HGQ time.

George climbed into the front seat, and in just a few minutes, we were ushered through the doors of a converted warehouse building by the West Side Highway.

The final cab of the evening found me and the porn star silent in the back seat. "Two stops," he said as we got in and without consulting me gave the driver my address. Then we were off, part of the swarm of urban bumble bees, the black and yellow schools that ruled the streets by night.

I stared out the window, thinking how he'd strut into that club as if he were the headlining act, even after we discovered the crowd was younger and more lesbian-heavy than I would have thought of a drag show. "The girls love Tricky," George explained. "Put him in a dress and he thinks he's a glamour dyke."

"Then why does he keep talking about his I.U.D.?" I asked. "Dress or no dress, he doesn't need an I.U.D."

Jason smiled at me. "Your thinking is too literal, Rachel. Gender is a more fluid thing, what do you think the internet is all about?"

George and Jason danced. RR surveyed the crowd, the way I'd seen him watch over the set, making sure he got his money's worth. So even-keeled was he as we moved from place to place, his bodyguard pose. I found it unnerving, particularly because I couldn't stop staring at the women dancing. I used to go to the Columbia dances with Jason and watch women dance together, but then I'd been detached, or at least believed myself to be. Now, I could barely keep up my sophisticated ennui when what I really wanted was to bump and grind with Shade on the dance floor, heated by the stream of the strobes, the flinging of bodies, and the thump-thump soundtrack that vibrated my feet and tingled my spine. A fluid thing, yes, but I was unsure of my motives, being with one and wanting the other.

It was an effort not to think of Shade, even with the strong, silent Republican sitting next to me, stretching his arm out behind him as if the cab were his coach. I leaned my head back into the seat, ran a quick loop through my mind: *He cups his hand around the back of Silver Ray's head and pushes it down to his lap. She feels around, unbut-*

tons his jeans, and there they are, her and that intimidating prick, up close and personal in the stuffy heat, the smell of animal hide.

I cracked the window. "Good idea," he smiled and I smiled and we must have looked like a couple of idiots; two yellow smiley faces in the back of a yellow cab. He was making me nervous, and when I got nervous I started feeling ethnic. Our cab had become a pumpkin, Silver Ray and her platform slippers had vanished, leaving me at war with my Eastern-European thighs, my Hymietown hair. Nothing like I'd been earlier, dancing with Jason, who kept saying how impressed he was with me. Such chutzpa, dating a porn star. The self-esteem it must require, not to mention the stamina. "You have no idea," I said, giving myself rare license to provoke. "I'm becoming an equal opportunity employer, too."

"Girls?" he said, and I darted my eyes around the room full of women, flaunting my ambivalence as if it were a diamond bracelet and not the usual cuffs around my wrists. I'd worked my HGQ, although I could feel it diminishing steadily since this silent cab ride began.

We pulled up in front of my apartment. "Thanks for coming," I said.

"No problem." He nodded, but made no move to kiss me or touch me or shake my hand even. Dejected, I clicked the handle, pushed the door with my foot, and climbed out. I didn't want to kiss him, anyway; I liked women.

"Listen," he said. "Do you want to go to Vegas tomorrow?"

"Are you serious?" I said, a bit shell-shocked. He couldn't kiss me goodnight, but he wanted to take me on vacation the next day.

"You still don't believe me."

"Okay, okay, I'm sorry, but no, I don't want to go to Las Vegas."

"Have you ever been?"

"No." I knew only what I'd seen in the movies: flashing lights and the green baize of gaming tables, sequined tights and tuxedos, call girls and comedians on the glitter circuit. I also knew it was where Neil lived, and that I would therefore avoid it.

"Well, you really should go," he said.

"Maybe I will."

"Just not tomorrow."

"No, not tomorrow."

"That's too bad."

"What is it with you and Las Vegas?"

"It's where I live."

Such simplicity again from the porno man—Rob Vaughn, with his conservative politics and cryptic smile. Where he lives. Sure, RR, whatever. I clicked my tongue against the roof of my mouth. "Well, viva Las Vegas to you then."

He laughed, and I liked the way his lips parted. Okay, maybe kissing him wouldn't be so bad, but no way was I making the first move. He would at least have to get out of the cab. I leaned my arm against the door, giving him one final opportunity to jump out or call me back. He didn't move. I sighed, "All right, I'm going in now."

He nodded. "See you around, Silver."

"Goodnight Mister…RR."

I slammed the door behind me, trudged up to my apartment where I kicked off my boots, slid out of my gown, and crawled into bed. There was something pathetic about lying naked in bed, alone. The wishful thinking and fantasies took over. If only I'd been more aggressive about him coming up. It wasn't Vegas, but I did have a couple of Elvis CDs to guide us through the land of make-believe. Yet, given my fantasy of choice, I would rather put on Chet Baker singing "My Funny Valentine," wound with the repeat button, the way I liked to listen to music: one song over and over again until I knew every word and breath and nuance. And Shade would be here with me, her body on mine, and...I felt sappy and weak. Lonely, too, planning the soundtrack for a scene that existed only in my mind. I turned on the TV: channel-surfed. The clock flashed three and I wanted to talk to Shade. A few minutes I wrestled the should-I-or-shouldn't-I concerns of late-night callers—number one being convinced that she had another lover with her—before taking my chances.

She picked up on the fourth ring, just as her machine was about to click on. "This better be good, Slivowitz," she said.

"I hate your caller ID."

"I have to be at the airport in a few hours."

"I'm sorry, I just wanted to talk."

"So talk," she sighed, and I told her about my evening, feeling particularly self-righteous since nothing had happened between me and the porn star, and we'd actually ended up at a drag show with a bunch of lesbians. Shade laughed, but wouldn't stop calling RR my boyfriend, choking on the word as if it were an aspirin tablet.

A brief lull in conversation found me staring at the half-lit walls. Beneath the covers, the fingers of my left hand tickled my stomach.

"What are you doing, anyway?" Shade said.

"What am I doing?

"Like, are you on the futon? In your PJs with a jar of Skippy?"

"Actually I'm in bed with the TV on. No sound, though."

Shade asked me if I was watching a porn film. I said no, then asked: "Should I be?"

"Sure."

I reached for the remote. *X-posure* already in the VCR, I fast-forwarded, giving Shade an overview of the plot, superfluous information about the characters and a few historical bits and pieces I'd picked up from Alexis. I slowed the tape at my favorite scene, the girl-girl action I'd practically committed to memory. "You want me to tell you what's happening?"

Shade laughed, said yes. "Well, Claire Blue has dark hair, blue eyes, and very red lips. Her neck is long, with thick jugular veins—"

"Please, Slivowitz! Not a coroner's report."

I felt my neck heat up. "Okay, her lover is taking her tongue and running it up the middle of her stomach, past her breasts...she's whispering something in her ear and they both look...I don't know."

"Horny?"

"Yes, that's a good word," I said, and prompted by Shade's questions, described the look in Claire Blue's eyes. I was overheating; my comforter felt like the full-body bib the dentist covers you with before an x-ray. I kicked it off and lay naked, my body shining like an x-ray star: Silver Ray in *X-posure* sweet-talking the sexy Shade, whose name was all the introduction she needed, honey. I was made for this business.

On screen, the action heated up. "She's back downtown again,"

I said, "with her tongue on her thigh and both her thumbs in her...I can't, I can't say it."

"Come on, it's easy. Just say it: cunt." The word sent shivers down my spine.

I laughed nervously. "Cunt."

"Very good."

"Are we having phone sex?"

"I think so, is that a problem?"

"No."

"Then go on, I'm all ears. And fingers."

"Are you...?"

"Uh-huh. Are you?"

"Not yet." I switched the phone to my left ear. I am a righty. "Okay, there we go, now where were we?"

"What are they doing?"

"Oh, remember, she's got her thumbs in her...you know."

"Her cunt, you can do it," Shade said.

"I can't, I feel stupid."

"Don't," Shade said. The rasp in her voice warmed my limbs. "You know how much I want you."

"No, I don't."

She sighed. "...umn, what can I say? It's been like forever. Remember the first day of the strike? I put the green M&M on your tongue, and I don't know, I just wanted to leave my finger there, and I hadn't felt that way in a while, at least not here in New York, and...oh..."

"No, please, don't stop," I whispered, and moved my middle finger on top of my clit.

"I'm...I'm getting all hot here for the record, but anyway, I don't know, when you kissed me...you know those kisses you feel in your chest? And *you* kissed *me,* I always thought I would be the one...and frankly, it scared the shit out of me, but since then it's all I think about. Baby, I want you. So much."

"I want you too." I fingered myself as if I were standing alone in front of the mirror, thinking: baby, baby, baby. No one had ever called me baby. A word straight out of the generic supermarket, it always sounded so patronizing in those rock-and-roll anthems by men, but coming from Shade's mouth got me all liquid. I had her repeat it a few times, then she followed with a play-by-play of what she would have done had she seen me in my black dress earlier. Her language was so crude and wonderful, a wire-tapper would have thought she was the one who'd been watching all the porno tapes. I would from that moment live to hear her say the word cunt in my ear, as she told me to add a finger and another until I was buried up to my knuckles and my wrist cramped. I knocked my head against the on-off button, accidentally hanging up the phone.

"Shit!" I pushed the button, got a dial tone. My call waiting beeped.

"You could give a girl a complex," Shade said.

"I needed both hands."

"Use something, go get a cucumber."

"Don't have one."

"A carrot."

"I don't eat vegetables."

"You really should, you're not getting any younger. How about a candle?"

"Too dangerous." I reminded her of the blaze of my Chanukah candles the night I'd kissed her and the three hundred dollars the vet later charged for the kitty colonics to flush the wax from Freddy's system.

"I guess you need my penis then," she said so seductively I was embarrassed by the image of her standing over me with a large strap-on and me, the big, fat bottom, craving her cock, begging for it. A flash of Tricky deep-throating his mike came to me. He'd said something like, "Fuck my pussy, you dyke bitch," and I thought it strange at the time, and even stranger now, finger deep in this gender fluidity business.

I lost myself in her words by the frosty glint of my TV screen. Closing my eyes, I stroked myself to the sound of her voice. I opened them, and there, as if set off in flashing lights, rested on my night table the toy pop-gun Mom had given me, its oblong shape and handle teasing.

I inched forward and quietly grabbed the gun, cocking the cork in place, sliding the handle into the body, slowly, so it wouldn't release. I slipped it in with a piercing jab, then the smooth swallow of my cunt and the feeling that the gun wasn't big enough, that nothing would ever be big enough. I moaned and said something like please.

"Oh yes, baby," Shade said. "Yes."

And those were the last sentences we spoke for a while, the static of our connection usurped by a moan & groan track to match anything in *X-posure,* with Shade throwing in the occasional, *oh baby, yes baby...*and I knew I was going to come as if it were the easiest thing in the world, as if it were the only thing in the world, and I didn't even care that her ear was so close to my voice when I did.

Our heaving subsided into laughter then silence, the peaks and valleys of social realignment. Finally, Shade said she had to go, it was almost time to catch her plane.

"Will you call me from home?"

"Sure," she said, and I saw myself waiting by the phone in the cold nights ahead. I would have to get a wall calendar and cross out the days until she returned. Or maybe I should just run a razor blade through my wrists and avoid the whole thing.

A few minutes later we hung up, both of us afraid to let go first. I pulled out the gun and it hurt, a piercing like loneliness. The gun moist in my palm, I read the word: Bermuda. My mother and her boyfriend went to Bermuda and all they got me was this lousy sex toy.

I pulled back the handle and popped it, shooting a few drops of fluid with the cork. My close up, my come shot, then the fading to black.

Porn Queen for a Day

After Shade left, I started taking long walks through Central Park, with big sunglasses and a scarf wrapped tightly around my head. I'd gone totally Jackie O, afraid even strangers might see the fire in me, the blush from my pop-gun that sent me out into the winter-wet air conjuring in my mind images of hiking boots, snow flurries at football games, and commercials for cold medicine. Today, I felt the perfect pitch of blue, like the weather. Or PMS.

I needed a hot dog with blood-orange onions. Never mind that I'd inhaled half a chocolate cake before leaving my apartment, I was hungry. These days my appetite was voracious, insatiable, fill in the adjectives. A hedonist's delight to fit my video box. Let's try ravenous: *Nothing was ever enough, at night she cried out for more... Silver Ray is "Ravenous!"*

So I kibitzed with my inner porn star as we hiked the urban tundra over to a hot dog stand. A man stood in front of me blowing smoke into his bare hands as the vendor ladled his hot dog with mustard and ketchup. It was short, the dog; probably less than six inches. At home, I'd been measuring objects with a wooden ruler, and then holding them against my stomach to see how high they'd get up inside of me. I needed some idea where twelve inches might land. A workable equation. The carrots, celery stalks, squashes, and cucumbers I'd purchased but had yet to eat all fell between six and nine inches. Bananas were about the same. The handle of my brush was five inches, the hammer ten, TV remote five, toothbrush holder six, cardboard kaleidoscope five and a half, pop-gun eight if you measured from the coconuts on the handle.

The man in front of me paid the vendor, and I ordered my little dog. Turns out, six inches was nothing, eight completely manageable, but only if it was as thin as my pop-gun. The other day I wrapped a condom around a nine-inch cucumber, but even greased couldn't get anywhere with it. Holding it against the toy gun I realized the vegetable was about three times as thick. Circumference was key. Pi times radius squared = R squared = RR = too big.

I ate my hotdog so fast the roof of my mouth was raw, then made my way to the skating rink to watch the ruddy faces go round and round, taking comfort in the other bodies braving this cold fish of a day. I stayed until I couldn't feel my toes.

At the Seventy-second Street exit, I came upon Santa Claus ringing his bell over a Salvation Army bucket. I smiled. He said, "Merry Christmas, baby," which I ignored. Nobody but Shade could get away with calling me that. "Are you on a soap opera?" he said even louder this time, and though I was tempted to say I was a porn star, I kept walking. "Bitch!" he blurted.

I turned around. "Excuse me?"

"You heard me," he said, his yellow-white beard attached crookedly to his lips, his muddy brown eyes full of blank rage. Something about his face reminded me of Kaminsky.

"How can you say that? You don't even know me."

"I know your type."

"You don't know anything."

"I know enough, you're a—"

"Don't you dare!" I screamed, alarmed by the menacing beat of my heart. A few people had gathered around us, apparently to see who had the temerity to raise her voice at Santa Claus. Naughty, not nice; I had to calm down. I leaned back a few steps and turned away.

"See, that's it," he taunted, shook his bell. "The way you move your head."

"What?"

"You know what."

"Look, do you have a permit or something? I'll call your supervisor." The knot of my silk scarf gripped my neck. This made me angrier at Santa Claus. He said something I didn't hear, then laughed so hard his cheap beard shook. Everyone around joined the playground choir. My chest cavity vibrated madly. Before I knew what was happening, I saw both of my palms stretch out in front of me and push against the pillow in his chest. He tripped backwards, and I kept pounding my fists against him, hoping to knock him over and shut him up. A thick arm grabbed me from behind. "Hey, settle down!"

I swung around and came face-to-face with the strong arm of the NYPD, the man's uniform as ridiculously blue as Santa's was red. I sniffled once or twice, wiped a tear from my eye, afraid that I'd flipped. The cop screamed away the crowd and led us toward Santa's unmanned coin bucket.

Had someone described this scene to me, I would not have recognized myself. Normally, I walked away from arguments, avoided scenes, and always backed down from physical contact. Whenever my parents started fighting I was the first to sprint from the room, and I spent too many hours hiding from my brothers. Once, when I was about ten, I did try to kick Neil, but like a masked goalie he caught my foot, and I fell flat on my ass. For weeks my walk was unbalanced and he called me a gimp.

That pain in my ass returned as I shrank further inside my skin. Santa brushed a few twigs from his suit and said, "She's fucking crazy, she hit me."

"He called me a bitch!"

"Okay, okay, I heard all I want to hear from both of you right now." The cop held out his hand in front of me, then turned to Santa. "Are you all right?"

"Barely, man," he said. "She should be locked up."

The cop nodded, yeah, yeah, then told me stay put while he walked Santa a few steps, whispering. I watched the cars speed to make the green light at Seventy-second, some zipping like luge racers through the park's curved entrance. Two girls dressed in little Eskimo coats ran past. "Mommy!" one said, "Tiffany killed one of God's creatures!" "Did not!" "Did too, I saw you smush it." The mother seemed oblivious, took each child by the hand, and dragged them across the street as they screamed: did not, did too, did not, did too....

I was suddenly embarrassed by what the cop must have seen, this diminutive mortal picking a fight with the season. She of the bugged-out sunglasses, and head wrapped in a babushka—by Armani, okay, but the *shtetl* connotations obvious nonetheless. I ripped the scarf from my head, setting my hair free. My ears burned, would soon be pink and pulsating like the rest of me. I was out of control, as if anything could happen; maybe this was what it felt like to be my mother.

The cop returned, said Santa wasn't going to press charges. "He's not! Oh, that's really great." Again, I felt the blood rush to my face. "He's a disgrace to that suit, the creep."

"Listen, lady, you got a problem with Santa Claus, call the North Pole. My advice to you is just go home."

I was too angry, the scene too absurd. So I tramped off, almost stomping on a framed picture of the Statue of Liberty, which kicked off a line of enlarged color snapshots lining the scarred cobblestones. A sign above them read: "Makes perfect holiday gifts." I wanted to take my platform boots and smash each picture. Like the Eskimo girl with a thing for smiting bugs, I would pulverize the World Trade Center, the Brooklyn Bridge, the Chrysler Building, the Museum of Fucking Modern Art. I hated this city sometimes, its slick skyscrapers and shiny streets; its tired, humble, poor, and weak all trying to keep up with the Joneses and Smiths and Slivowitzes, our voices blending a dirge despicably modern, like the big-bang of a holiday blockbuster, a virtual mushroom cloud over the all-new, brilliantly digitized Times Square. So modern, so now, twilight's last gleaming. New York was falling apart with progress, going down on me, and all I wanted was to go home and masturbate. Use my fingers, the pop-gun, anything to silence the raving lunatic who'd pitched a tent in my cunt. But I was not crazy, not like my mother, not crazy, not like my mother.

I clenched my fists deep inside the pockets of my wool overcoat, and fought the mournful winds all the way home, where opening the door for me in his tight, synthetic-fiber, stripe-down-the-side doorman pants was Yossi the Israeli. Not to be confused with Yuri the Ukrainian who had a terrible acne problem, nor Max the gaunt Bronx native who could tell you where every celebrity in the area had lived or died. Yossi was my favorite. He smelled nice and had good teeth. But before today I'd never thought about dragging him by the balls down to the laundry room and screwing him in a *Sensurround* sort of way: hard, bloody, and foreboding. My desire these days took two genres: *X-posure* and *Sensurround.* Call it a yin-yang thing. A battle of milk and meat.

Yossi pressed the elevator button for me and I noticed his fingers, thick and probing. Those fingers could ravage me...*Silver Ray is Ravaged!* A bing and the elevator doors opened. "Have a good day," he smiled, the moment gone.

Upstairs: the mail. Solicitations, magazines, bills, which seemed to arrive more frequently than they did before the strike, and one mailing envelope with Shade's handwriting still reeking of indelible magic marker. I felt inexplicably happy, silly as a showtune. It had been a week since our conversation, and part of me was afraid it was all a dream, the sex-talk, the coming, her *oh, baby, I want you so much!*

Not fast enough did I cut the envelope and amid the newspaper shavings remove a Ziploc bag full of green M&Ms. My body swelled as if my internal organs were being pumped. I stripped down to my tank and underpants, sat cross-legged on my bed, and pulled open the bag. I rolled a smiling green M&M between my thumb and forefinger. Popped it in my mouth, sucking until the coating melted and I tasted the sweet chocolate inside. A tear escaped the corner of my eye: you little sapster. I stuck my entire hand in the bag and with my fist squeezed and released.

Green fingers sticking to the phone, I called Shade in Atlanta, never so excited about talking to anyone in my life. The way she said my name when she picked up, as if I were the only person in the world, made me feel drippy again. She told me to hold on, there was someone on the other line. I sucked another M&M, fearing the day I might be on the other end, dissed for caller number two. She clicked back. "So is it true?"

"True?"

"About the green ones."

I laughed. "I wouldn't know, I'm completely premenstrual. I had a fight with Santa Claus in Central Park."

"How Scrooge."

"He started it."

I told her about the fight, and she teased me. But before we could go any further she said she was on her way to the mall. Shopping with mother. "Seems we can only talk around the spirits of Donna and Calvin and Christian."

"I like mine when she's on Demerol."

"Are you okay?" she asked, her voice so present I thought I might start sobbing. Instead, I took off my tank.

"Yeah, I'm okay. Are you okay?"

"I think so. Is it cold there yet?"

"Freezing."

"Then you'd better stay inside. I'll call you later."

"Goodbye, Shade."

"Merry Christmas, baby."

Her words left me stroking my pussy with an M&M, enough to taste myself on the candy. Freddy scratched at my toes. I nudged her away with my foot, touching myself with one hand and eating the M&Ms off of my stomach with the other.

The phone rang: I was screening. Mom's voice came, faintly, something about borrowing my jeep. I reached for the toy pop-gun she'd given me and imagined she'd put a spy camera inside. She was watching me masturbate. Her voice fragmented—*you said you'd be here over the holidays.*

...oh, yes.

—Lorraine's gotta be by her doctor.

I saw Aunt Lorraine's face and wanted to scream...no! The gun moved faster, fucked me deeper, stomping and smashing Mom's voice, breaking the whole damn world...ouch!...my toe...I kicked the cat and was coming and scared and coming and sad and coming and utterly humiliated. I smelled myself on the clammy sheets. That's it. I was through with this business. I reached for Freddy, but she mewed angrily, threw her tail up in my face. "I'm sorry," I said, talking to my cat, again. Each day took me one step closer to cat-lady land. I knew I had to get out of solitary, yet everywhere I went

I dragged my smelly bed along with me, wearing a sign that marked me worse than a scab. I was a daughter of Onan.

"Go ahead, try them on," RR said, a dare of course.

We were behind the shoji screens sectioning off Mistress Wanda Lynne's dressing table, perusing her wares—the standard handcuffs, whips, nipple clamps, masks, paddles, etc. What had caught my interest was the pair of thigh-high patent leather stilettos. About twenty-four inches high.

"Come on, they're not ready yet," he goaded, and in his voice lay my claim to ambivalence. As much as I wanted to try on the boots, I didn't trust him. But the way he smiled at me, nothing short of provocation, inspired my Silver Ray recalcitrance. I sat down on a folding chair next to him and removed my own platform boots. Fortuitous, I hadn't done laundry in weeks and had to dig up a pleated, black mini-skirt I hadn't worn in years. *You are not honest, Slivowitz; you knew he was back from Vegas when you dressed this morning.*

Shade ghosting me, I removed my platforms and lifted one of the shiny thigh-highs. It felt smooth against my fingers and smelled of shoe polish. "It's like a heel upgrade," I said, conscious of RR's eyes on my feet as I slid them one after the other into Wanda Lynne's boots, pulling up at the thighs so the leather gripped tightly. His staring aroused me, for despite his pleas to the contrary, I couldn't separate him from his porn star identity. He was all sex. The frivolous and seedy kind. The kind they advertised in the back of magazines and on cable TV.

"You gonna walk or what?" he said.

"Hold your horses." I balanced myself on the back of a chair, took a few steps. It was as if I were walking on stilts. Awkward and defiantly nonerotic. I kept thinking, please don't fall, please don't fall. But I'd always been a fast learner. A few more steps and I sailed with the curve of Silver Ray's hips, the swagger of her triple-X ass.

"Not bad," he said.

Not bad? I was pacing in front of him like a Madison Avenue hooker, and he says not bad. Bastard. I handed over the reins to

Silver Ray. She took a step toward him, then another. Close enough to touch, she teased, pivoted, the back of her thighs in his face. She leaned forward, keeping all of the weight on her legs, and felt him move closer, his breath on her ass.

A quick second, the shift of my eyes, and there was Mistress Wanda Lynne, yellow-blond hair glimmering against her black satin cape, the chunky soles of her white combat boots lifting her almost six feet in the air.

"Excuse me, but what the fuck is this?" Her eyebrows swept up her forehead. I slipped forward, would have fallen on my face were it not for the dressing table. As it was, I knocked a riding crop to the floor.

"I...uh...I was just—"

"You're wearing my boots!"

My mouth opened, but no words came out. I was counting on RR to speak, but he just sat there. Smiling, I think.

"Jesus Christ...Alexis!" she screamed, then ranted. "These are my things, this is my work. I don't go to your job and go through your things! You wouldn't catch me trying to do your job!" Alexis pulled back the screen, took a quick survey. A few of her minions came running behind her.

"Wanda?" she said, and I knew I was in trouble. Alexis Calyx frightened me more than some tatty dominatrix, more than a belligerent Santa Claus or the entire NYPD for that matter. It wasn't that she was my employer, but that her opinions had started to count.

"Who the fuck is she? She's wearing my boots!" Wanda Lynne shouted.

"I was just trying them on," I protested.

"You can't do that, who said you could do that?"

"Okay, look, she's not going anywhere with them," Alexis said. "Rachel, take off the boots."

I sat down and yanked the left boot by its five-inch heel. "No!" Wanda said, hands on hips, cape flying out at the sides. She looked like a superhero. "Don't pull from the heel! It doesn't matter, they're ruined."

"What are you talking about?" Alexis said.

"I can't wear them if someone else's feet were in them. It's a bad omen, ask anybody. This is so unprofessional."

"They're just shoes," RR said.

"Shut up, Robbie," Alexis said. "But, you know, Wanda, this is a little extreme."

"Oh you think this is extreme? Watch."

She turned and started packing her equipment, the back of her cape flailing left and right with each aggravated movement. By this time, what seemed like the entire cast and crew of *One in the Hand, Two in the Bush* had descended upon Mistress Wanda Lynne's dressing table. Nobody uttered a word. A few chains clinked and zippers locked, every sound amplified as if the set had been miked. Wanda's stilettos bound my feet in day-glow cuffs.

As with yesterday's run-in with Santa Claus, I had difficulty placing myself in this scene. I hated being the center of attention and, usually, did whatever I could to blend into the background. This wasn't so odd for a journalist. I was great with people one-on-one, could lure confessions out of the most stoic of subjects, and I had no trouble walking into a room full of lawyers, cops, or junkies as long as I knew I wouldn't have to participate. On the other hand, editorial meetings were torture, dinner parties a nightmare. The one time I'd mistakenly accepted an invitation to speak in front of a group of journalism students, I spent a couple of weeks vomiting, my body reaching unprecedented levels of dehydration, before I had to cancel the engagement. Sam suggested hypnosis. I think I told him to piss off, or words to that effect. Funny, I wasn't nauseous now, though all eyes led inevitably toward my feet. I was more nervous about Alexis.

Finished with her packing, Wanda stomped off the set. Then, as if a pause button had been released, confusion ensued. It was the only scene left to shoot, and they needed a dominatrix, Alexis said she wouldn't compromise. Call Wanda and apologize, someone said. Offer her more money, new boots, anything. "Get another mistress," said Alia the directorial ingenue.

Alexis looked apoplectic, as if the suggestion had been for her to walk across burning coals. "On Christmas Eve?" she said. "Where am I going to find a dominatrix on Christmas Eve?"

"This is New York," said a young man I didn't remember and would have remembered because he had a row of about twenty metal rings in each ear.

"Fine, okay. Fine." Alexis swung her arms overhead. "You think you can get someone, by all means, go right ahead, whatever you have to do, go for it."

They walked off. Others paced, making frustrated faces, offering the same suggestions over and over again. Listening to them, I felt guilty and feared being banished from the magical kingdom. Another casualty of the Alexis Calyx ghostwriting wars: Rachel the porn star wanna-be. She was fourth, fifth if you included the sister. I bent down to remove the offending thigh-highs.

"Hey, why don't you use Silver here," RR said, forcing me to look up at him. "She's wearing the shoes."

"What?" Alexis snarled, and I wanted to smack the sanctimonious smile from his face. I couldn't believe he said that after he'd made me try on the boots, the traitor.

"Of course, sure, she could be," said Claire Blue. It was the first time she'd addressed me other than a quick *bonjour* and slight slip of the lip, so much like her take-me mouth in *X-posure* it always made me blush. I could barely even look at her, let alone think about acting in a movie with her. As if I could act in any kind of movie, with anyone. I fidgeted when Rowdy pointed his video camera in my direction, and Silver Ray, too, was a behind-the-scenes kind of gal. It was part of her shtick, the camera-shy porn star. But silence had fallen on the set, everyone staring at me as if the suggestion that I stand in for Mistress Wanda Lynne were not the height of absurdity.

"Oh, no," I nodded fiercely. "I can't do it, no way."

"Yes, but, why not?" Claire Blue looked at me, and I made myself hold her gaze. Her ink-black hair framed her face; her eyes were perfectly blue, depressed but regal like the weather, like blue M&Ms. Stage fright or not, I might do the scene if I got to kiss her afterwards. "You see yourself with the shoes, that's all," she said. "I am the one really who is doing everything. You just say the words, hold the whip, tie me around."

"The shoes do fit," said Bob Florida, a blond military type also in the scene.

"Yes, they are good," Claire Blue said. "She looks beautiful too, eh? A little fear makes a woman more, I don't know, sensual I think."

"Absolutely," RR said.

"Um...thanks," I stammered. "But, I don't think so."

"Hello, over here, objection!" Alexis shouted. All eyes turned to her. "Can we get back to the planet earth now?"

While I was thankful for her clarity, I was also insulted. She didn't want me in her movie. I wasn't good enough, pretty enough, sexy enough.

"You should listen to Claire," RR said. "She's French, she knows about these things. Haven't you read *Story of O?*"

"Get out, okay? Just get out!" Alexis pointed her cell phone at RR's face. He rolled his eyes.

"You're overreacting, Alexis," he said.

"Don't patronize me, just get off my fucking set. You've done what you wanted, so get out."

"You serious?" he glared at Alexis, his prune face meaner than I'd ever seen, taunting and belligerent. A look of panic seized her, the olive tones draining from her skin as if someone had drawn them from her cheeks with a hypodermic. But only for a few seconds. She managed to shake it off and walk toward RR. The rest of us were immobile, a captive audience. "You bet I'm serious," she said. "I'm sick of you trying to sabotage me, and I'm really sick of feeling guilty about your career."

"You're forgetting whose movie this is."

"No, I won't let you do this anymore!" She swung her phone like an epileptic conductor. I was afraid she might hit him with it. "I want you out of here and I don't give a shit if you pull your goddamn money. I shouldn't have taken it in the first place."

"You can't do this without me," he said.

"I'm serious, get the fuck off my set, Robbie. Just leave me alone!"

He pursed his lips dismissively and laughed. Then he did something so audacious, so vulgar, so fucked-up and aggressive....

He winked at me. As if we'd been in collusion! Mortified, I wanted to disappear inside of Wanda Lynne's boots. But I felt gigantic, awkward, and inflated with anger. I could have pummeled him the way I'd taken out Santa Claus. He was such an asshole. I took a deep, calming breath, trying to convince myself nobody had seen him wink or that maybe I'd imagined it. RR turned back to Alexis, and they stared, the set so quiet I could hear Claire Blue fidgeting next to me. I held my breath until finally, like my mother leaving the Thanksgiving dinner table, RR strutted out of there as if he were the innocent victim of a witch hunt and the rest of us the condemning masses. The worst part was I wanted to storm out with him.

When he was gone, Alexis turned to me. "Meet me out front, I need some air. And get rid of those boots, please."

"What should I do with them?"

"I don't care, just get them away from me, I never want to see them again."

Claire Blue helped me slip the boots from my feet. I put on my platforms, my coat, grabbed my bag. She rolled each of the thigh-highs from the bottom, then stood up next to me. She was short, maybe five feet. On her back she gave the impression of being a towering figure.

"Take them, they look good." She handed me the boots and smiled softly. I couldn't believe this was Claire Blue, the woman I fast-forwarded to whenever I watched *X-posure.* I wanted to tell her that I'd seen the film a few times, thirty or forty, not too many; tell her that I'd been coming more than ever and she was somehow part of it; tell her that I might make myself available to do the scene in my bedroom, away from the cameras. Maybe I could be her rehearsal partner.

But, ultimately, all I said was, "Thanks."

She gave me a card for her one-woman show at The Performance Warehouse in January. "You can write something perhaps."

I slipped the card in my pocket, buried the boots deep inside my bag, and left the sound stage. Alexis was waiting for me outside. She wore a tight leather coat over her skirt with the high slit, a knit skull cap, and sunglasses—all black. I felt as if I were cavorting with a fashionable corpse, only I was the one being led to the gallows.

We walked to Tompkins Square; it was another chilly, wet afternoon, the clouds a radioactive gray. I felt overwhelmingly sad and guilty. Worse, every time I tried to apologize, Alexis brushed me off with a cold glance then picked up the pace. I wished she would yell at me or reprimand me, let me repent at least.

Alexis stopped at the dog run, and we hung our arms over the fence, both of us looking forward. She sighed, shaking her head at me. "Little Rachel Silver from Bay Ridge," she said.

"I'm really sorry," I said again. A small furry dog humped the leg of a golden retriever, as if he were hanging on the only way he knew. It took me back to the porn set, Wanda storming off, those burnished boots declaring it my fault. The wave of fear that had washed over Alexis, destabilizing her in a way I never imagined possible, if only for a few seconds. I felt miserable.

"Are you going to fire me?" I asked and immediately felt my heart leap.

"Do you think I should?"

"No."

"I'll take that under advisement."

"So in other words I'm sitting in limbo."

"Look," she said. "You've put me in a strange place. I don't want to lose you. You're smart, you laugh at my jokes, and I think we understand each other."

"But?"

"You're a lot like me, too curious for your own good."

"Are you talking about him?"

"You won't listen, that's clear."

Her words pierced my chest like a stiletto heel. I was a ball of self-loathing and trickery. That we both knew RR was behind my trying on Wanda's boots made my betrayal more poisonous. I vowed silently not to see him again and wanted to convey this to Alexis. Maybe then she would console me the way she'd comforted Tessa Torpedo my first day on the set. She pivoted toward me, and I felt hopeful. But I couldn't get beyond her dark sunglasses.

Again, we looked out at the dogs running happily, chasing sticks and balls, barking, growling, and crotch sniffing. Maybe they knew more than we did about communication. There was something to be said for sniffing people out before getting too close.

A cold wind settled between us. My fingers started feeling brittle inside my leather gloves, and I wished I were at home in bed. The ring of the cell phone made me jump. Alexis grabbed it from her bag, and a conversation ensued. She said "Fabulous!" a few times, while I shifted my weight from leg to leg to keep them from freezing. Apparently, they'd found a dominatrix willing to work all night if need be. Alexis was pleased.

She slipped the phone back into her bag, raised her eyebrows. "Okay, let's do a little experiment, which one is the Rachel dog?"

"The what?"

"Don't pretend you don't know what I'm talking about, I'm getting tired of this. The Rachel dog? I say it's that big black sheepdog." She directed my attention to a silly dog lounging beneath a tree, panting as she watched the rest of them play. It was a good guess, the doggy-voyeur with her hair flopping in the wind. I figured she was making fun of me.

"I think I'm more that one," I said.

"Which?"

"Over there."

"The German shepherd?"

"No, the little one by the fence." Though embarrassed by my canine self, I pointed to a spunky fox terrier who kept picking fights with the bigger dogs and running away. She wanted to play, but was too shy or too scared or too pristine. In the hierarchy of the dog run she was a fence-sitter.

Alexis nodded; she saw it, too.

"So which is the Alexis dog?"

"I'll let you decide. I've got to get back and see this thing through."

She left me at the dog run more confused than I'd been when we first entered the park. But before I left I did see the Alexis dog. An elegant Weimaraner who sashayed back and forth with a cadre of smaller dogs at her feet.

I stayed in bed two days, not touching myself, not turning on the television, not answering the telephone, not thinking. Indolence of such magnitude was no easy feat. I had to silence my answering machine, swallow a few Tylenol 3s, and arm my CD switcher with Billie Holliday, Barbra Streisand, Patsy Cline, k.d. lang, and Madonna ballads. I had lost all interest in men, musically. The women spoke my kind of suffering; among them thousands of tears had shed.

Then, just before New Year's, I got my period and opened the blinds to an eyestrain of sunshine that twinkled the streets as if they'd been glazed. A winter day so beautiful it was almost obscene. I showered, dressed, and drove out to Bay Ridge.

Mom and Hy had already left for their spa near Atlantic City. Rowdy claimed to have a lead on a job he didn't want to mention for fear of jinxing it. Whatever it was it kept him out of the house. Meanwhile, I settled into my old room, which didn't feel like my room at all. Only the diplomas on the wall, a World Book Encyclopedia set, and my creaky twin bed remained from childhood. The rest of my past had been obliterated.

Not Aunt Lorraine, though. We played endless games of backgammon and gin rummy like the old days. I mixed chocolate egg creams and prepared salami sandwiches, dousing them with bright yellow mustard and cutting them in quarters, the way she used to do. We watched a lot of television, mostly entertainment shows and off-beat sporting events. Aunt Lorraine had taken a particular liking to monster truck competitions.

On New Year's Eve we sat together on her bed waiting for the ball to drop. I was fine until I saw all of those people in Times Square so obliviously cheering on time when I wanted only to hold it back, bowdlerize eternity. I zapped the sound, suggested another game of backgammon.

"I beat you already three times," Aunt Lorraine said. "Besides, I'm feeling good. Maybe I could get in the chair and go outside."

"Are you kidding? It's freezing out there, supposed to snow again."

"Then how about we go downstairs and watch from the living room."

Grateful for anything that might take us from the televised reverie, I said okay. I detached the IV unit from her arm and put a new gauze bandage around the tube, impressed with my ability to pretend I wasn't grossed out by the blood, the black-and-blues, the yellow-green of her skin. Messages from the body, as unnerving to me as cries from a newborn.

Aunt Lorraine grabbed my arm, and I immediately recognized the soft grip of her hand. She was the only person I could place by touch.

Downstairs, I helped her onto the couch and drew back the living room curtains. I sat on the windowsill, toyed nervously with the curtain string. A thin layer of snow glazed the ground, tiny flakes dancing beneath the streetlights. My old block, sheer and sparkling, got me every time. I wanted to cry, but kept a tight lip.

While I did feel something like a stewardess on a crashing plane, I experienced a side of myself I barely recognized: that prosaic maternal instinct. Being with Aunt Lorraine put me as much in touch with Eve as Alexis Calyx had in the past weeks let me commune with Lilith, for Eve was the first earth mother, Lilith the prototype of every sex-positive feminist. I'd heard Lilith was wild and uncontrollable, and she liked being on top, an obvious sign of maternal deficiency. So Adam complained to God, who banished Lilith to the tainted status of succubus, paving the garden path for Eve. Why was it that in the beginning man was one and woman was two? Her self divided along the lines of how she fucked: for purpose or pleasure.

And people wondered why women were so screwed up, why all the eating disorders, clinical depressions, self mutilations, sexual hangups, and suicides. But I am being reductive. My journalistic training says avoid generalizations. Specify the statistics. Three concrete examples of anything and you've got a trend. I flashed on my mother, my aunt, and myself: women were screwed up about sex.

Aunt Lorraine exhaled loudly. I looked at her sitting on the couch like a child, her feet barely scratching the floor.

"You look sad, hun," she said.

"Me? Nah."

"Oh bullshit. It's New Year's, you should be out having fun, not stuck inside with an old lady."

"I hate New Year's. And for your information I'm not stuck here, I want to be here."

"You're a terrible liar."

"I'm serious, anyway, I wanted to ask you," I felt my heart speed up, my armpits get sticky. "Are you still watching those movies?"

"Oh, some. Rowdy's been getting them from the video store. No offense to your friend Alexis, but she should make her films trashier, that's what gives 'em their kick."

"You sound like the writers at *Porn Star News.*" She laughed, and I thought the best defense was a humorous offense. A line like that could have ended the conversation and Aunt Lorraine would have been none the wiser. We'd never talked personally about sex before. But the urgency of her situation was changing the way we communicated, giving language to topics that were always taboo. Still, my heart drilled against my rib cage as I ventured. "But when you say kick? Do you mean...?"

"Oh, come on now."

"Are you talking about, you know," I bent my head down, hid inside my right elbow. "I mean, do you feel...oh boy, this is hard."

"Just a little bit tingly, who doesn't?" Aunt Lorraine answered. I couldn't believe she used the word tingly. "But mostly they bring back memories."

Memories? All they'd given me recently was an addict's craving, less from want than need. Were her memories of sex steeped in such desperation? Or was she being more literal? My mind jolted. Aunt Lorraine was a showgirl. A Betty Page co-star. Maybe she'd owned a brothel. I wasn't sure if I could handle this.

I hid behind a few giggles. "Okay, what are you talking about?"

"I had my time, you know."

"Right, but memories? That's pretty hardcore stuff."

"It's just like dreaming, like remembering the ones you sometimes want to pretend you never had. What you do with them is your business, and in my day a lady kept to herself, didn't go shooting her mouth off all over television...oh, you're so surprised? I always told you about my sweethearts."

"True." My heartbeat settled slightly. Whenever Aunt Lorraine returned from weekends in the Catskills, she regaled me with stories of Saturday night swing dances, high-brief bikinis, and flowered bathing caps, men named Izzy, Mo, and Herman. But as with her stories of their escape from Poland, she revealed little emotion. It was as if she were a commentator packaging the facts for airplay, her point of view left behind in a mountainside bungalow.

A place I could see, now, in Aunt Lorraine's face, rheumy-eyed beneath her Yankee cap, yet almost glowing. This woman knew all that Alexis Calyx knew.

"When you said sweetheart, I thought love, not sex." I turned my head to the window to check on the snow, but also to avoid looking at her. It was beginning to hurt too much too often.

"Best when they come together."

"Were you in love with any of them, the sweethearts?"

"Once or twice, but they ended."

"Don't they always," I sighed.

"Not always. Romance, the touchy-feely business, it's a big circle, finishes itself off like your movies. Love's what's left."

"But you said—"

"Even when it ends it stays."

"I don't want you to die," I blurted out, still staring outside, knowing that if I turned just slightly I would start bawling for sure.

"Honey, I'm hanging in as long as I can, but this is no life for a lady." The snow fell faster, in big, cottony flakes. "I'm getting tired," she whispered. "So tired."

I fell asleep at the foot of Aunt Lorraine's bed that night and woke up while it was still dark. I'd done this many times as a child, but never remembered the room being so quiet. My heart did a quick sprint. I jumped off the bed and put my hand over her face. Slowly, I felt my palm warm. Then, as my eyes adjusted to the dark, I deciphered the expand and contract motions of her stomach under the white sheet.

I kneeled down beside her, eyeing her smooth, almost translucent skin, her fallen eyelids, so big and purple, eyelashes like pieces of wet thread strung together.

We were getting closer, so I set my sights small. If only we could make it through the winter, not have to battle the icy roads. I lifted the heavy afghan from the chair next to her bed, draped it over my shoulders, and walked to the window. Dark and dreamy, yet so desolate it made me shiver. I pulled the afghan tighter around my body, smelled a lingering scent of the hair creme Aunt Lorraine no longer had any use for. She'd knitted this blanket back in the days she was never caught without a colorful roll of yarn in her lap. As a child I'd tried to help her, but, like Mom, could never get it quite right. I had no patience for the sedentary.

I left the window, stretched my limbs across the carpet next to Aunt Lorraine's bed like the faithful little pooch I was. No matter what I could or couldn't do in the dog run, I felt okay at home. Until home started slipping away.

I couldn't sleep, but didn't dare move, remained still until my thoughts became indistinguishable from my dreams. Like dying, or maybe something else.

The Broadway Episode

Arriving at The Movie House ten minutes late, I spotted a braided Shade wearing a red cocktail dress and sipping a frothy drink through a straw. I was nervous, but relaxed a bit when Shade upon seeing me broke into a stream of relentless smiles. It was her smiling I'd missed these last few weeks, the way my own face responded with burning cheeks.

I melted into the seat across from her, took off my gloves, my coat, unraveled my scarf. Her eyes perused my torso, encased as it was in the dress I'd bought earlier, short and black with a low scoop in the back. "You look all grown up," she said.

"You look like you did when I first met you."

"My mother." She rattled her extensions then held up her hands. "I had three manicures, okay. Three. I have no nails."

I took her fingers in mine. "They're so glossy."

We finger-frolicked until the waitress came. I dropped Shade's hands and ordered a Coke. Her toe nudged my left leg underneath the table. I looked out the window. Evening with its hopes and promises glowed in front of us, streetlights blaring frosty white spots upon the nicely dressed tourists, little pieces of recycled glass sprinkling down the jet black pavement. Even the taxi cabs looked elegant.

"I don't want to go," I said.

"We have to."

"Why?"

"Because."

"Because why?"

"We just do."

"And what if we don't?"

"Not an option."

"But it's your first night back."

"A couple of hours, that's all. It'll be a hoot."

The waitress brought my Coke, and we sat silently, Shade's foot tickling the back of my knee. I stared as if taking photographic stock of her eyes, her lips, the tiny cleft of skin on the right side of her nose, the result of a jet skiing accident that left her nostrils slightly lopsided. It said she was a bit of risk-taker. Hovered the voice of my dead father, the lay photographer: *You have to watch, to look, to eavesdrop on the face; hundreds of stories come and go in a minute.*

I wanted them all; but there wasn't time.

We bundled up and stepped outside, breathing heavily through the thick winter air. Though I endeavored another round of pouty "I don't want to go"s, I was soon following Shade through the gold-plated doors to the theater on Fourty-fourth Street, poised to see the new Mark Tannon play, a love story about a couple of veteran journalists set in Saudi Arabia during the Gulf War. Not that I wasn't impressed the TV newscaster had the spunk to write a play, but this benefit preview for the Newspaper Guild and their friends—the latter being anyone who could shell out the five-hundred-dollar ticket price—made me nervous. You had benefits for diseases or starving children, not newspaper reporters. Having just left Aunt Lorraine this morning, I was perhaps morbidly biased, but in the hierarchy of suffering I would say we were down there with landlords who felt abused by the vestiges of rent control.

Yet in this magisterial lobby with its gold leafing and marble, the tuxedos and sequined gowns roved, shiny leather shoes sinking into the plush red carpet. Gigantic tear sheets were propped up on easels, stories culled from newspapers throughout the country.

"We're national news?"

"Damn, Slivowitz," Shade pulled back my arm, stared as if she were frightened by me or for me, I couldn't tell.

On our way to the bar, I recognized a few faces, media media looking for quotes, gossips mingling about in couture clothing, a few tailed by buglike TV camera crews. The local news and entertainment channels taking tape all gravitated toward the banner plastered across the foyer: WE'RE WITH YOU STRIKING REPORTERS.

Shade went to get drinks; I leaned back against the wall, watched the slippery smooth party-goers tout a plastic chic. Their privileged vitality made me want to scream. But everyone else was eating it up. Arrogant waiters delivered hors d'oeuvres of chicken kebab, beef cubes, red-pepper shrimp, tiny skewers of shitakes, tomatoes, and yellow peppers. On the buffet table were cheeses, breads, grilled vegetables, pasta salads, cold meat platters, falafel balls, humus, baba ganush, and couscous—Gulf War food. Enough to make the mouth water, the stomach bloat benefit-style, like the kids in UNICEF posters.

I couldn't eat anything, I felt too queasy. Shade brought me a Coke. In her other hand was a pink drink in a martini glass. "Cosmopolitan," she said, and took a shrimp from a fashion model with a platter. She dipped the shrimp in hot butter sauce, and, navigating the strategic difficulties of balancing food and drink, shoved it in her mouth. She wiped the corners of her lips with a cocktail napkin. I wanted to kiss her.

"Shit, there's Hamlish, I'll be right back."

"Don't leave me!" My lower lip quivered. Shade touched my arm with her shrimp hand. "What?" she said, her lips and eyes widening simultaneously. "Are you really that socially challenged tonight? You look so beautiful." I felt as if she'd spilled hot shrimp butter all over my body. It was warm and liberating, like peeing in my pants as a child.

I turned away, found myself drowning in a sea of black backs with snatches of the rainbow glimmering in between. Then, like an apparition slowly materializing in the physical world, Jason appeared in front of us. I had to shift into neutral.

"Isn't this so very very?" he asked. Shade let go of my arm. Jason noticed. I could tell by the drift of his eyebrows, the lilt in his voice. I'd given away too much that night at Ethan's. He knew he'd stumbled upon a little scene. I knew he knew. He knew I knew he knew and so rolled the unspoken wheels.

"Yes, indeed, the hottest ticket in town tonight," he said. "I had to whore my front page to get on the list. They wouldn't even let me bring a guest."

"Do we get the cover this week?" I said.

"Not you, dears, striking as you are. We only want Tannon, that is if his play isn't the piece of royal garbage I suspect it will be."

"One can only hope," Shade said. "Listen, I have to go and catch Hamlish."

"That rodent...why?"

"A little thing called work."

Jason put his thumb and forefinger to his goatee, stared at Shade. "Miss Teesha Marie, why didn't I think of it before? My movie editor quit last week." They talked about what Shade might do for his magazine. I sank further into the wall. Underneath the big banner, the Mayor gesticulated pompously, a bouquet of microphones like bulbous vibrators at his lips. I resented him being here only slightly less than I resented being here myself.

Shade's voice soothed me somewhat, though I wished it were coming directly in my ear like our night on the phone. "You guys aren't union right?" she said.

"Are you joking? We thrive on maintaining utterly sadomasochistic relationships between talent and management."

I shifted my weight, twirled the plastic straw around my empty Coke glass. I barely realized I was stabbing my ice cubes until Tony joined us. "I think you killed one," he said. He was wearing a tuxedo that pulled too tightly around his stomach and carrying a pink drink like Shade's.

"You won't believe who I just bumped into, and I mean literally bumped into," Tony said. "I was going down the stairs just as she was coming up. She being the one and only Kim Mathews, so I said, 'Outta my way, TV bitch.'"

"You didn't?"

"Okay, I just smiled."

"You should have told her that chiffon in January is a no-no," Jason said. "How can I possibly trust her news judgment now?"

Jason kissed my cheek and announced that he was off to "do" the foyer. Tony took out his pouch and drizzled tobacco shavings into a piece of cigarette paper. "I heard she had her lumpectomy filmed," Shade said.

Tony eyed her quizzically. "Who?"

"Kim Mathews. They're going to air it during sweeps."

Though Shade and Tony seemed mildly shocked by this, it made sense to me after watching Rowdy with his third eye tracking Aunt Lorraine these past months. But the Mathews lump was benign, it had been all over the news; Aunt Lorraine's was deadly. Thoughts of sickness and death seemed incongruous among the cocktail-hour liveliness. I turned my attention to Shade and Tony, who were gossiping about the rest of our colleagues, many of whom had paraded before us at some point in the last half hour. *Did you hear McKneally got picked up by the* Post? *James was indexing textbooks. Carrie had a breakdown and went on Prozac...*Listening to them, I decided my ghostwriting job was a striker's Horatio Alger story.

Shade sent Tony to the bar, and he returned with three pink drinks. I didn't want mine, but thought it complemented my dress. I took a few fruity sips before the bell rang in the first curtain call.

"You're strikers?" a fresh-faced blond woman cut into our circle. She was about my height, had her hair pinned on top of her head with a glittery bar, and wore an expensive-looking business suit. I noticed the reporter's notebook sticking out of her jacket pocket.

"Gerri Michner," she said. "From the *Post,* I just wanted to get —"

"The quote du jour," Shade said. "Here goes: we're mad as hell and we're taking it up the wazoo. You can have that word for word, it's Teesha Marie Simpson. S-I-M-P-S-O-N."

"I know who you are."

"Now, now," Tony interjected. "It's been a distressing time for all of us, not knowing where we stand, who to trust, so I have to say it's pretty cool that everyone's come out to support us."

"And don't forget Mark Tannon," Shade said. "Bringing the experience of TV journalists to Broadway, it's so Ben Hecht."

Gerri Michner looked confused, made a few scratches in her notebook. I imagined her writing down the name Ben Hecht with a big question mark next to it. It was what I would have done. She looked up and caught me eavesdropping.

I was transfixed by her, so green and aggressive, the way I'd once been. A part of me longed to be back there with her, to be a reporter again and not the subject, to believe I was on the side of truth and not a *cause celèbre*. I felt a cramp of nostalgia that made me angrier than anything I'd seen tonight.

"How old are you?" I asked.

"What?"

"I bet you just graduated from some fancy journalism school?"

"In June. I got the internship at the *Post* and they hired me, like right after the summer."

"You really want to be part of this gossip mill?" I said, thinking of Aunt Lorraine and her gauzed lymph nodes, the orange stains on her nightgown, how easily the energy drains. "Look at them, all the nice clothes and three-hundred-dollar haircuts, they're all so self-serving. Why don't you go and follow some insurgent rebels? Do something on health care."

"Not everyone's a truth-seeker," Tony said.

"I cover the media." Gerri Michner glared at me. "You of all people should know this is news, unless you've forgotten what that is."

The nerve of that grasshopper, so smug, so active. "What exactly are you saying?"

"Just that you're not working."

"Looks like you need to brush up on your research skills, I happen to have work."

"Oh, yeah, what?"

Shade put down her empty glass, tugged at my arm. "I think it's time to go inside."

"I'm ghostwriting an autobiography for Alexis Calyx."

"The porn star!" Tony said.

"Feminist pornographer, she makes films now," I said. Gerri Michner's nose wrinkled. "What's the matter, are you one of those anti-porn women? You think it's all degrading? That women shouldn't like it, too?"

Gerri Michner scribbled something in her notebook, looked up. "It's a tired argument, but you don't think pornography's degrading?"

"Women have a right to pleasure, and I'm not talking about running through the flowers like a feminine hygiene commercial."

"And we know how pleasurable that is," Shade said, locking her arm around mine and attempting to push me away. The second curtain call sounded.

"Did you know she was doing this?" Tony asked Shade.

"Of course she knew," I said. Shade's chin dropped, and her eyes blew wide as a cartoon character. "What? I can't say that?"

"Then neither of you have any concerns about her working for a pornographer?" Gerri Michner said.

"Concerns?" I said. "What kind of concern—"

Shade jabbed her elbow into my stomach. I lost my breath and spilled the remnants of my Cosmopolitan on the carpet. "Dammit!" I screamed. Shade twisted her head around as she tugged me away. "The answer to your last question is: no comment."

A few feet away, Shade let go of me with an angry shove. We glared at each other. Around us, the hum of voices, the buzzing of bodies scrambling to find their seats. I suggested we go inside, but Shade just stood there. "I don't understand you," she said. "You know, this isn't a game and these aren't actors playing out your little fantasies. It's the goddamn New York media!"

"You're such a hypocrite, you're always talking about how open you are."

"Yeah, for real. Not to titillate some dumbass reporter!" Her words echoed in the now-empty lobby. She walked to the coat check. I followed silently, trying to recall if in all the years I'd known her I'd ever seen her this enraged. The golden doors shut behind us, and she continued screaming as if our few minutes of silent bundling had kindled her anger. How could I shoot my mouth off like that? Did I take anything seriously? Didn't I see that I'd put us in jeopardy?

"By telling her about my job?" I broke in, my breath visible in the cold, dark night. "Look, pornography is a part of life. If people can't deal with it, that's their problem."

"Of course it's a part of life, but it's private."

"I can't believe you're saying this."

"Jesus, Slivowitz, I'm a black woman, okay? Not to mention one who likes to sleep with other women. You know how this industry is, even though nobody will admit it because it's New York and we're all supposedly so enlightened, but I can't afford this shit!"

I leaned back, felt my hair pull against the cement wall. It pinched almost as much as the disappointment in Shade's eyes. She shut them, tilted her head up: story #14—the what-am-I-going-to-do-with-you face. Her eyes opened, she sighed, and I still felt lousy. "See, this has been my problem all along, why I was wary of kissing you that first night. You're playing, you don't know what you want."

"I want you."

"One minute, sure, and then the next minute you're going to a party with that porn star. It's like we're all part of some experiment."

"It's real, this...you...." I couldn't finish. Instead I looked down and saw two pairs of feet in stockings and pumps. My clothing had grown up faster than I had. I looked at Shade, hoping if I locked eyes with her she would see I wasn't playing. Her face softened slowly, and I sensed she knew, or maybe the cold was getting to her. Either way, she tugged me by the sleeve over to Broadway to hail a cab.

I woke up to Shade's bare back, the darkness outside reminding me I'd probably only drifted off a few minutes ago. She slept soundly, barely moved. I don't know why, but I'd pegged her for a midnight mumbler, lip-twitcher, and limb-wanderer.

Meanwhile, I couldn't keep still in my own bed. I thought about getting up and taking a magazine into the bathroom, the only space in my apartment with a door that shut, but I didn't want to leave Shade, not even to float a balmy bliss toward sleepyland. I was afraid of waking up and finding her gone. So I remained as if in a sentinel box, memorizing the perfect triangle of Shade's back, her head with its tight braids slumbered against my peach pillows. I wished she would wake up and take me in her arms the way she did last night after the hours we'd spent on the couch, both of us in our ridiculous cocktail dresses, talking until our eyelids curtained and voices cracked, talking, sometimes as if we'd known each other forever and other times as if we'd just met.

We kissed in the dark and it felt like an old jazz song. We kissed with our clothes on, long, soft kisses with our legs intertwined and dresses hiked up to our hips. Finally, I unzipped her, she unhooked me, and we were half-naked, me wearing nothing but a pair of black pantyhose, and Shade in matching bra and underwear, black with lacy red flowers—a bit Victoria's Secret I'm afraid, but we'd come from a benefit. We crawled beneath my comforter and kissed some more. It was me who pushed further, unsnapping her bra and burying my face in her breasts. She patted my head affectionately first, then harder. I felt her grab my hair, pull my head up to her chin. "Not yet," she said, and I wanted to cry or scream or smack her. She held me tighter, whispered, "I don't want to be drunk."

That I understood. She needed it to be real as much as I needed to prove it to her. So we held each other, fighting the same soporific divide that now had me watching her back, dueling with my weary eyelids, slipping back into the black hole of morning.

The ringing telephone jostled me. I'd fallen asleep again...shit! At least Shade hadn't left, I could feel her stirring next to me. She reached her hand back and I squeezed it. The voice of Alexis Calyx flooded in between us: "Rachel, I must speak to you immediately. I'm a bit disconcerted about the situation you've created."

Shade turned over, leaned against her elbow. We looked at each other and immediately knew what Alexis was talking about. "Guess we're not the only ones who missed the play," Shade said.

"I cannot have reporters calling my home," Alexis continued. I was about to pick up, when Shade grabbed my wrist. "We don't know what anything says yet, we need the paper, the information."

She got up and stood at the edge of my bed. Alexis hung up. I stared at Shade who was smiling a half-mocked, *You bad girl, Slivowitz.* I'd apologized a lot last night while we were talking on the couch, but still couldn't scrape the embarrassment from my skin.

Shade went into the bathroom, leaving the door open behind her. She turned on the shower. I drifted back to sleep imagining her, then woke to her footsteps. She was wrapped in a towel, her body scented with lemon soap, her mouth tasting of toothpaste. "Do not even tell me you used my toothbrush," I said.

Story #27—the guilty child routine. Was I supposed to reprimand her? Put her over my knee? I was the guilty one, the bad kid.

This reversal made me a little uncomfortable. "I warned you, baby, no half-assed shit," she said, obviously pleased that she'd spent the night in my bed. She kissed me fiercely, then, rubbing her hands together like a fruit fly, stood in front of my closet. "Now...your clothes."

We suited her up in a pair of hiking boots, faded jeans, and a ribbed turtleneck, which I pulled over her bare shoulders and smoothed down at her waist. Before sending her out on the newspaper run, I kissed each of her nipples for good luck. The wool tickled my lips.

I took a quick shower and erased Alexis' message from my answering machine. I was tense, but energized, feeling groovy enough to switch my stereo from public radio to hardcore disco. Moving to the rhythm of the boogie, the beat, I straightened the magazines, videocassettes, and remote control units on the coffee table, swept the tiles around the kitchenette, wiped down the counter, swished a little bleach around the toilet bowl. Cleanliness demanded urgency now that somebody was looking.

I'd just finished the Cinderella routine when Shade came barreling in. She dropped a few plastic bags. A bagel broke free and rolled along the floor.

"You lost your bagel."

"Oh, just you wait." She shed my snorkel jacket, dropped it on the couch, and paced, flipping through the paper for Gerri Michner's column. I lowered the music, sat down on a kitchen stool. "Okay, I hope you're ready," she said and started reading. "Despite an angry despondence among reporters gathered at the Mark Tannon benefit last night, one reporter on strike had a confession to make: 'I happen to have work,' said Rachel Silver, a midlevel reporter—"

"Midlevel, what the fuck is that?"

"That's nothing...midlevel, covering the courts, blah, blah...'I'm ghostwriting the autobiography of Alexis Calyx, the feminist pornographer,' Silver said. 'Like Alexis, I believe women have a right to pleasure, that women can like porn, too.' Silver's colleagues, as well, were shocked by her new employment. 'I had no idea she was working for a porn star,' said former city desk reporter Tony

Dibenedetto. Arts reporter Teesha Marie Simpson, also on strike, had no comment."

My heart sank hearing Shade read her own name. We exchanged a quick glance, and she read on, a comment by one of the union leaders about how I was collecting strike pay and therefore should have reported *any* outside employment, "particularly something that might compromise the moral standards of the union." Next came the off-the-hook statement, that a spokesperson from Zipless Pictures would neither confirm nor deny whether Alexis had officially hired a ghostwriter, although Gerri Michner did manage to dig up a lackey who admitted to seeing me hanging around the set asking questions. "People are always passing through," said the employee who wouldn't give his name. "You never ask who anybody is because you don't want to offend the next big star or someone who might be throwing money our way, that kind of thing."

I tugged at my mousse-hardened hair. "We're almost through," Shade said, and read the grand finale, how whether or not I was officially on the Calyx payroll, I was certainly towing the pro-porn line. "You want to talk about morality here," I said, apparently. "Look around you, these people are all so self-serving, just like the anti-porn women."

I jumped up from the counter. "Did I say that? I couldn't have said that, it's totally out of context."

"Well, sort of."

"She's saying I called everyone there anti-pornography."

"No, she's saying you called everyone self-serving. You only called *her* anti-pornography."

"Not the way she said it." I turned my head away, close to tears. Shade grabbed my flailing arms by the biceps.

"Baby, I'm sorry," she said, the fear in her eyes summoning last night. As from a scratchy newsreel, the images rolled forward: Gerri Michner's face, how badly I'd wanted to show her up, trumpet my Silver Ray liberation as if it were a badge of honor. My jaw shook, and I felt as if a marble had lodged in my throat. The phone rang. Shade and I shrieked, jumped backwards. "Good morning, you lovely loose cannon," began Jason's message.

"Oh god," I said. "I am such an idiot."

"Don't worry," Shade said and lifted the telephone, Jason's voice sailing through the speaker a few seconds before she shut off the sound and ringer. Watching as she fit the phone underneath my bed, I was thankful Gerri Michner had left Shade out of it, that the fears about her reputation had not borne out. If for no other reason than to have her sitting on my bed, looking as if she might smother me with tenderness.

"Come here, my little loose cannon," she said, there, on my tousled sheets, in my clothes, looking like love should, equal parts desire and consequence. I felt every breath crawl through my heart as I walked toward her amid the faint roll of the drum machines. A Moog, a melody, and those digitally mastered cries of passion and dreams and shaking it, baby, shaking it because when you dance it's all about making love, isn't it?

Shade leaned back on her elbows. I fit myself in between her legs, her hands parted my bathrobe. Soon I felt nothing but her fingers.

So evening came, and morning came; it was the first day, and then the second before we left my apartment. We walked the wet streets, as if we were inside of a bubble, one of those scenes you shake and the snowflakes swirl. It wasn't snowing yet, but the air was heavy, the sky a mist of gray guncotton.

We bought coffee in paper cups and continued on, going nowhere. Shade stopped in front of a vendor hawking hats, modeling a few, as I sipped my coffee through a crack in the plastic lid. She chose a black, knit cap, the kind worn by urban thugs on television. "Are you planning on turning over a candy store?" I asked. She smiled, said the hat made her feel tough. But she was more of a sap than I was. When we passed the multiplex just as the feel-good movie of the season was about to begin, she begged me to go inside.

"Come on, Slivowitz," she cocked her upper lip at me. "Ever made out in the movies?"

I didn't have to answer. I'd always been urbane about moviegoing, arriving early to be Coke-and-popcorned by the first preview, and barring all communication once the lights went out. On occasion, I'd even shushed a peanut-gallery commentator or two. But there I sat kissing in the back row like a clumsy adolescent, though not my adolescence—for I'd never even kissed a boy until I was eighteen years old, and never would have imagined that all the boys I'd kissed since would be obliterated by one woman in a dark movie theater.

We were feeling good, so much so that we skipped out before the movie ended and ran back to my apartment, forgetting that we'd originally come out for food and toilet paper.

Home again, as if we'd never left the bed, I was overwhelmed by my craving for Shade, my longing to bind her hands and feet so she couldn't leave. Yet, whenever I tried to express these feelings without sounding like the mildly neurotic and needy adult I was, my language retreated to the vapid patterns of pornolinguistics.

"I'm waiting for this to blow up," I said, moving my leg beneath her until I felt her on my knee.

"What?"

"This you and me against the world thing."

"Don't say that."

"It can't last."

"Yes it can," she said, and despite the barrage of phone messages from Alexis, union leaders, Mom, Aunt Lorraine, various friends and colleagues, and, that first day, a few scavengers from the media hoping I might be a loose cannon for them as well, I believed her. I would have believed anything she told me with her body on mine, her fingers slipping inside me and teeth biting my nipples, a little bit hard, which I discovered I liked. Though I couldn't come, I felt closer than ever, beyond it even, the way the graze of a finger can in the right circumstances be more intense than a grasp. Still, there was the dark-continent part of me that believed our relationship would not be fully consummated until I had an orgasm.

Day four, alone in the shower, I gave in and masturbated. Though it wasn't the climax I'd wished for, I came in about two seconds. It was insidious, a litmus test that left me feeling physiologically defective. A sexual misfit. Not like Shade who could come when I fucked her, but only if I used two fingers at about a forty-five degree angle so the base of my hand hit her clit, and even then, only after she'd gotten off once already some other way. This kind of specificity amazed me. Clearly, Shade's was a sexual history spawned by trial and error, along with a few creative lovers all of whom I'd become insanely jealous of; jealous because they'd been with her, but also because of the things they'd done together. None of the men I'd been with even liked being on their backs.

In all fairness I couldn't blame them entirely. I never said what I wanted, what I liked, and through my frustrated silence I'd grown contemptuous of their easy orgasms. I'd lorded my frigidity over them as if it were a sacred cow. But it ruined me sexually.

"I understand now," Shade said. It was day six and I'd finally confessed that I was indeed troubled by my not coming.

"What?"

"The other night, at the benefit. There's just no letting go for you, is there?"

"I guess not." I looked up from the couch where I'd been clipping my toenails. She was sitting at the counter in my bathrobe, drinking a glass of orange juice and not-reading a magazine.

"It's all inside," she pointed to her temple. "That's the real sex organ, the rest is just friction."

I pursed my lips, returned to my clipping.

"No, really. We'll figure it out."

Let her hope, but I knew better. People who came easily never understood this, how it felt to be perpetually on-the-verge, revved-up and good-to-go, but then you're going and going and going and suddenly everything shuts down, like someone flicked a switch in your head. Whatever you do next is inconsequential, you've passed the point of no return. Bottomed out. Sometimes when I hit bottom, I became so dejected and angry I couldn't speak for hours. Other times, I could pretend I'd actually come, feeling sated enough by wet sheets and a lover's arms. With Shade it was mostly the latter.

She took the nail clipper from my hands and sat down next to me. "There's something I want to ask, don't be mad, but—" she giggled so I knew it wasn't serious. "In your closet, I saw these...these boots."

"They're the real thing, straight from the dungeons of Mistress

Wanda Lynne." I explained about the mishap on the set, yet in the telling it seemed as if the entire day had been lived by someone else. Silver Ray, perhaps.

At Shade's request, I took out the boots, and together we inspected them. "They're sort of scary," she said.

"I don't think so."

"Put them on." She smiled, and within seconds was helping me into the thigh-highs I'd inherited because that idiot Robbie Rod had cajoled me into trying them on when he must have known it was bad karma to wear a dominatrix's boots without asking. That day I'd been devastated, but balancing around my apartment for Shade I wished I'd thanked him.

"Take off your underwear," Shade said, and I did, the sun making waves through my dirty blinds, and it was naughty and illicit, as if we were slumming in a dive bar in the middle of the afternoon. But if in the boots I'd felt like a whore with RR, with Shade I was a woman, or I accepted some idea of femininity that had always felt like an act with men. I liked being sexy, I liked her watching me being sexy.

We danced naked and I was suddenly tall. She put me in her lace bra and spun me around. "There, now you look like a porn star."

"I have way too much pubic hair."

"Let's get rid of it."

"You serious?"

She nodded, cheeks dimpling foolishly, but I knew she was indeed serious. She said she'd always wanted to shave a woman and, at that moment, she could have said she wanted to have a threesome with a goat and my response would have been, "Let's find a petting zoo."

An occasional advocate of the clipped bikini line, I had the necessary accoutrements. Scissors. Shaving cream. Disposable razors. Vitamin E capsules and aloe vera lotion. Shade draped a towel over the toilet seat and sat me down, spreading my patent leather legs. She picked up the scissors and my thighs caved inward. I had this fear of sharp objects near my pussy, especially when they were in somebody else's hands.

"It's okay," she said. She kissed the top of my clit, stroked me with her fingers and already I wanted to scream. I leaned my head back, felt the pull of my pubes, the cold metal of the scissors, and then, a tense snip. My eyes shut to the clip of the shears, the hum of Shade's voice.

When I next looked down, my pubes were tightly buzzed; sort of prepubescent, sort of in-the-Navy, yet caught between these shiny leather lampposts. I almost liked my own body. Shade smiled, filled her palm with shaving cream and my heart beat wildly.

She started shaving from the top. The back of my neck tingled, and I had to bite my tongue to keep from whimpering. I could feel my legs shaking the closer she came to my vagina. "Trust me," she said, two fingers spreading my lower lips so she could get in further with the razor. "I was always really good at shaving the balloon. It was my favorite booth at the town fair. I won prizes."

"You're such a little suburban girl."

"I never said anything different, everyone just assumes I'm from Brooklyn or wherever. From the 'hood, as it were."

"I'm more from the 'hood than you are."

"Exactly, but it's like that's the past I should have had."

"You can have mine if you want."

"That's very kind of you...can you move your left leg up a bit...there, that's it." My right leg slanted against the sink as if I were a contortionist so Shade could get underneath. In flooded visions of losing my balance and sacrificing my clit to a disposable bic. No coming, ever. Not even the hope of it. I shivered, felt the muscles in my stomach contract.

"Relax," Shade said, as if she'd read my mind. She softened the scrape of her razor, stopping every so often to stroke me with her fingertips. I felt them so intensely, the opposite of relaxing.

She pulled back, tapped the razor against her chin. "I'm wondering, maybe we should leave the hair on top."

"You're the stylist."

"Here." She tilted a hand-held mirror toward me.

"Ugh, it looks like a moustache."

"Our customers are mad for it, we call it the Charlie Chaplin."

The little black hairs sneered above my cunt. Bald, I could handle, but these few molded strands reeked of a slow, uncomfortable death. "More like Adolph Hitler," I said. "I hate it, take it off."

She grabbed my chin in her free hand, kissed me, then returned gallantly to her shaving. When she finished she rubbed me clean with a warm washcloth, and I felt pampered, cared for in a way I'd never experienced.

White fluorescents streaming, she dropped to her knees in front of my bald vagina. She licked me slowly, so tenderly it hurt more than the pull of her razor. She pushed my legs further apart, fingered me. On her knees, she was licking me and fucking me and I could feel it this time, feel it for real. I was thinking please, please, please...but I lost it again, was soon ambushed by those familiar frustrations. There was just no letting go. I lifted Shade's head. "You're all wet," she panted. I started sobbing.

We fell down on the cold bathroom floor, Shade's arms mainlining relief as I wailed maniacally. I said I was sorry for not coming, and she said it was okay, it didn't matter. "I was almost there, I swear it." I hiccuped, and she held me, for hours it seemed. I'd never cried in front of a lover, never cried so deeply with anyone before, not even that day in Kaminsky's office when I realized I was losing Aunt Lorraine for good. Such emotion frightened me, felt more foreign than my shaved vagina.

I longed only to comfort her back, be good to her, but my own feelings were so overwhelming they left me mute and immobile. Ultimately, I was afraid I'd failed her and would always fail her, because I couldn't give her what she wanted. I couldn't give her everything.

Darkness eclipsed my studio, offering a night and day contrast to the two of us in this light-bright bathroom. "I'm starving," Shade said.

"I know, but I can't move."

Gently, she lifted me, put her arms around my waist, and hugged me.

"Sorry I ruined your fantasy," I said.

"You didn't ruin shit."

"It's not what you wanted, it should have been sexy."

"It is, Slivowitz," she whispered, her breath mingling with my ear lobe. "It really is."

I don't know whether I believed her or not, but the words felt right. As did her body on mine, stumbling from the bathroom and collapsing back into bed.

Good Morning Heartache

On the seventh day, Hy called and said that Mom and Aunt Lorraine had been admitted to the hospital. Nothing to worry about, both were doing fine, he repeated a few times before telling me what had happened. They'd been watching television the night before when Rowdy barreled in screaming. "Get the doctor, man! She ain't breathing right."

Mom and Hy followed him upstairs where they found Aunt Lorraine wheezing uncomfortably with her eyes closed, the sight of which caused Mom to drop. Rowdy called an ambulance. When Mom, after they'd roused her, complained of heart palpitations, they put her in the back seat of Hy's Cadillac and followed the ambulance to Sisters of Mercy Hospital, whereupon they both were admitted. Aunt Lorraine had broken a couple of ribs, Mom, they suspected, was suffering from exhaustion.

I got out there as quickly as I could, all things considered. Orienting myself to the world after stowing away seven days was difficult enough without having to leave Shade. I dropped her off on my way to Brooklyn. We stared out the windshield for a while, holding hands over the stick shift.

"I wish I could go," she said, finally.

"I know, but...you know."

"I know."

Our language had become a pyramid; it's foundation vast and firm, we barely needed words anymore. Yet as soon as we parted, I feared the last few days had been a lie. I felt disconnected, utterly exposed. As if cast from the garden, I was doomed to walk the planet naked, all eyes on me, taunting me for my shaved cunt, my watching porno films, my sleeping with another woman, everything. Like Lilith, I was banished and horny and alone.

These visions of sprites and spirits were magnified at Sisters of Mercy Hospital. Most of the nurses wore crosses, and biblical scenes adorned the walls. Hy had to hang his coat over the painting of Jesus across from Mom's bed. "I couldn't stand him looking at me," she said.

She was fully dressed, face painted. Hy said all the tests had come back negative and she was about to be released.

"I'm glad you're okay," I said.

"I'm telling you, Ray, you should have seen it," Hy said. "They all come in here and bow down in front of him."

"In front of who?"

"Him, the big guy, in the painting. So, I try to take it off the wall and guess what? It's nailed down." He laughed hysterically, was joined by Mom. I must have looked confused. "Nailed down," he repeated, waiting for my response with his mouth agape.

"Jesus...ooops!" Mom laughed, covered her lips with her fingers. It amazed me how animated she became when she was the patient. Normally, she couldn't walk into a hospital without fainting.

"Don't you get it?" Hy said. "They say the Jews crucified him, but they got him nailed to the wall."

"Oh."

"Forget it, she won't laugh at Catholics," Mom said.

"It's a bad joke," I said.

"Look at her, acting all high and mighty after she tells the whole world about the filth she's involved in."

It took every ounce of self-control I had to ignore her comment. I walked to the window, tried to find my jeep among the cars in the parking lot. Already I was antsy and wanted to get back to Manhattan.

A doctor came in and had Mom sign her release forms. Hy lifted his jacket from the Christ painting. I half expected to see the devil jump from the frame. But he was just your average Jesus, a long-haired guy in a bathrobe. I followed Mom and Hy back to Aunt Lorraine's room where Rowdy was videotaping Aunt Lorraine and Kiki talking about *Days of Our Lives.*

After a quick powwow, during which I barely spoke, we decided to have lunch. Then I would come back later for the meeting with Aunt Lorraine and her oncologist. She'd asked me to be there, and I'd said yes, resigning myself to the fact that I would not be leaving Brooklyn for a while. Though I felt a bit resentful, I swallowed it as I leaned over and kissed Aunt Lorraine's cheek. "Buckle up, hun," she said.

"What?"

"Your seat belt, can't be too careful."

I took a deep breath, laughed. As much as I sensed her words were coded, I adhered to them when Rowdy and I settled into my jeep for the short trip to the diner. We got there first. By the time Mom, Hy, and Kiki arrived I'd memorized the descriptions of the various Belgian waffles and Rowdy had eaten all of the rolls in the bread basket.

"Our chauffeur here made a wrong turn," Kiki said.

"You said right, I went right," Hy said, and that was only the beginning of his bickering. He sent back his soup. Then, after he'd dropped his spoon on the floor, he demanded another, saying it was filthy anyway. Finally, when his burger came, he cut into it with a knife and sneered as if he'd discovered a hair or fingernail. "Say, young lady!" he bellowed at the waitress. His voice pierced my ear drums. A few heads turned our way, the waitress rolled her eyes, walked over.

"I said medium rare, this is still bleeding," Hy said. "Take it back and cook it, would you?"

"Everything's gone downhill here," Mom said.

"When you been here before?" Rowdy asked.

"They're all the same."

I couldn't care less about Hy's food, the downswing in service at diners, nor whether Mom's emergency visit was covered by her HMO. I tried to remember if I still had health insurance while on strike, but couldn't. This upset me, the not remembering. My thoughts clouded over with Jesus Christ and his downy nimbus,

Aunt Lorraine and that feeding tube in her arm. "It's a nice hospital, very clean," she'd said upon my arrival. I remembered touching her shoulder, biting the inside of my cheek until it stung.

Kiki nudged my arm. "You gotta eat, Rachey, you're getting too skinny."

"I'm not hungry," I said, though I was starving. I couldn't remember the last meal I'd eaten. But after two bites of my chicken salad sandwich I felt nauseous. It was like my not-coming, no matter how deep the craving I couldn't satisfy it.

"Can I have your fries?" Kiki asked. I passed my plate to her.

"Wait, wait," Rowdy reached out his hand and grabbed my sandwich. "You don't want it, right?"

I nodded no.

"Rowdy, give me her pickle," Mom said.

They devoured my food before ordering dessert. I moved my sunglasses from the top of my head back over my eyes, drank another cup of stale coffee. I didn't speak again until I stood up and, leaving them at the diner, returned to Sisters of Mercy Hospital to meet the cancer doctor.

Two zero-degree days passed before Aunt Lorraine could leave the hospital. Rowdy and I borrowed Hy's Cadillac and found her as feisty as usual. Insisting that she was no invalid, she eschewed her wheelchair, instead clinging heavily to our arms as we walked through the hospital corridors and out into the savage winds.

It took a while to get her upstairs and settled into bed. I sat down next to her, a pang creeping from the pit of my empty stomach into the back of my throat. It was a combination of fear and anticipation that I imagined as a ball constructed of thousands of rubber bands.

"You'll stay tonight," she said and, though I'd been hoping to get back to Manhattan and see Shade, I said of course I would stay with her.

"Good, because it's time we talked serious."

"Serious?" The ball in my neck started bobbing.

"Open that drawer over there." She pointed to her side table. Inside the top drawer were two containers filled with tiny orange capsules. The labels read Seconal. I removed one, the pills clicking as I opened the child-proof top. A couple of pills I examined in my palm. They were so bright like the psychedelic orange from a black-light poster or neon orange road signs with big Helvetica letters: Warning.

Alongside the pill bottles was a stethoscope, its base coiled neatly around the earplugs. There were also a few books on assisted suicide, including Kaminsky's self-published "how-to" guide, and a stack of business cards tied together with a broken rubber band. A few of my own bands snapped. I slammed the drawer shut.

"I can't do it," I said.

"You only think you can't."

"No, I can't. Isn't that why we got Kaminsky?"

"He's here if we need him, but we won't."

I stood and began to pace, exhaling loudly. It took every ounce of strength I had not to bolt out of there. "I can't go back to the hospital," Aunt Lorraine said. "Understand that, please, just understand that. This is too much already. I'm not living right; I'm stuck in this bed all day...I go to stretch, I break two ribs...I can barely pee on my own."

Her voice filled the room, a checklist of crippling pains and ailments. She spoke of everything I already knew, everything I would have expected, but I'd been duped by Jesus and the kindness of a few nurses. Her doctors, too, had been dangerously upbeat.

"Honey, please," she said.

I leaned against the bedroom door, stared at her. A red bandanna covered her bald head, and I thought of my own hairless state, the discomfort it had been wreaking inside my underpants.

"Does your head itch?" I asked.

"Not so much." She touched a couple of fingers to her head as if reminding herself she had no hair. "It's soft, like baby skin. Want to feel it?"

"Okay."

I walked to the bed and helped her untie the bandanna. Bald, she looked stalwart, a monument to individual bravery, or so I kept telling myself, avoiding her eyes, trapped as they were within the purple sockets of a once fully fleshed face. Gone were her ruddy cheeks and bushy eyebrows, lost was the rubious glow of her lips. As painful as it was for me, it must have been devastating for her. I don't think she hated anything as much as she hated being sick.

Though I felt a little creepy, I put my hand on her head. It was as soft as she'd said, just like her hands. "Look, promise me this at least," she said. "You won't let them put me back in the hospital."

"Okay," I said, my palm on her velvet pate as if I were swearing in a court of law. Behind my back, however, I crossed the fingers of my other hand. I wasn't sure I could do what she wanted. I knew only that I had to get out of Brooklyn.

I left at the crack of dawn to meet Alexis Calyx at a Midtown post-production house. Exiting the Brooklyn-Battery Tunnel more than an hour ahead of schedule, I decided to stop by Shade's apartment. Had I a cell phone, I might have called ahead. I felt funny stopping by unannounced, that was more Shade's style than mine.

I parked directly in front of her building and stepped outside. The air had a bounce to it, the kind that kept you dancing on cold winter days. Or was it, perhaps, the grave pounding of my heart that had me shuffling my feet and blowing steam into my cupped leather gloves? I pressed the buzzer. There was no answer, so I pressed again. Finally, came her voice: "Yeah?"

"It's me."

A few garbled words floated from the speaker.

"It's freezing, Shade. Open up."

She buzzed me in. I yanked open the two sets of doors to her brownstone and inside found her standing in the doorway of her first-floor apartment. She was barefoot, wearing jeans and a tank top, and looked as if in my figure she'd seen a ghost. I wondered if I'd carried death all the way from Brooklyn.

At the door she whispered, "Tina's here."

"What?" The mention of her name set off the ball of rubber bands in my neck.

"Trust me, it's nothing."

"Nothing?"

"I'll explain later."

She led me inside, and like an idiot, I followed. Tina Macadam sat on the futon with her legs crossed. Her maroon hair was darker...wet. She casually smoked a cigarette.

A nervous Shade kept her words breezy as she introduced us, though the situation told each of us more than we'd wanted to know. I sat down on a lounge chair next to the futon and unbuttoned my pea coat.

"Have you recovered from the Tannon benefit yet?" Macadam said, shooting straight for the heart.

"It wasn't a big deal," I shrugged it off.

"Right, she's very resilient," Shade said, pacing. "Did you want coffee?"

"Apparently so are you," I snapped at Shade, then looked down. On the hard wood floor lay my ribbed turtle neck, next to it her flowered bra: signs like glowing Seconal pills. I wanted to wrap the bra around Shade's neck, tight.

"Everyone makes mistakes, Slivowitz," Shade said. Upon hearing her use that name, I went soft for a second, felt as if we could boot the intruder and spend the morning making love.

"You said it," Macadam said. "They arrested a bunch of people for tipping a truck the other night."

"No!" Shade said, and a conversation ensued about the enervated spirits on the picket line. Shade brought me the coffee I didn't remember asking for. I took a sip, then put down the cup. Source light showered through the window, turning curlicues of dust and highlighting the dirty veins and ovals sprawling like mammoth vaginas upon the almond floor. Shade and Macadam talked on, their words sounding like Swahili; I felt more in synch with the cranking and whining of the radiator. Trapped in Shade's baking apartment, there seemed no tidy way out of this predicament. That I worried about having a scene only fueled my self-loathing, but I was getting sick of scenes. Still, I could not sit here making small talk, pretending our sensibilities so modern they precluded jealousy, ourselves so evolved we might fall into a threesome as any porn film would have scripted it. One of those happy coincidences, like the goddamn Dominos man at your door.

Macadam's voice ripped into me. Her head swung backwards

and I imagined her coming. She could come and I couldn't. Maybe they'd even come together; I was the intruder. I felt sick to my stomach, had to get out, but again feared breaking their conversation. *Do it, Slivowitz, just get up and leave!*

I pulled back the sleeve of my pea coat, felt a bead of sweat escape from my temple. "Um...I've got to be somewhere," I said, and it wasn't a lie. Shade turned to me, her face a wide-eyed signal I tried to decipher. Story #41—*flagrante delicto.*

I stood, said a quick goodbye to Macadam. Big of me, I thought. Shade bounced up from the couch, said, "Wait!" I pulled open the door and fled. She ran after me in her bare feet, screaming my name.

"Slivowitz, damn you!" She caught up and pushed me against the side of my jeep. "I told you it was nothing."

"It was nothing or nothing happened?" She rolled her eyes, looked down. "Jesus, Shade, your bra was on the floor."

"She showed up totally out of it."

"So you had to have sex with her."

I turned away, banged my fist against the roof of my jeep until I felt my palm sting. Shade spun me around. "It's not what you think, I totally shut down."

"You know, I'm sitting there thinking, why is Shade in a tank top, why is what's-her-name's hair all wet? And there's your bra like a goddamn disco ball."

"I'm trying to untangle things, and keep it all healthy."

"Oh, get out of here with that. Life isn't healthy, that's the biggest scam." She let go of me. I looked down, caught her nipples poking out of her tank top, and craved her naked body on mine. She must have been freezing, though she tempered it. As if she were impervious to trivialities such as the weather.

Resisting the urge to hold her, I broke away and walked around to the driver's side. I fit my key in the door. "You're missing the point as usual," she said.

"The point being?" I looked over the roof at her.

"I'm in love with you, you jerk."

"You've got an interesting way of showing it."

"At least I can say it. I love you and I fucked up, okay? And it wasn't even a big fuck up, nothing really happened, so I'll live with it."

"How nice for you."

"Hey, it's not like I haven't been patient with you," she said, and her words confirmed everything: Tina Macadam could come and I couldn't. I felt as if I'd had the wind knocked out of me. Shade's face dropped. "Oh god, I'm sorry. I didn't mean that."

My heart raged inside my coat, and I no longer felt the cold. A few people passed, double-taking upon noticing Shade in her tank top. She didn't budge, kept looking at me until I started feeling guilty when I was the one she'd just taken down. I opened the door to my jeep, almost tore it out of its socket I was so angry.

"Slivowitz, I—"

"Spare me."

"I'm the idiot now."

"I really have to go." I climbed into my jeep.

As I drove away, in my rearview mirror I saw her hugging her arms around her body. Barefoot in the dead of winter. I should have told her to go inside and warm up, but not with Tina Macadam there. I slammed my horn a few times, started running red lights.

The morning rush passed as if it were a video game. With every street came a new challenge: red lights, green lights, flashing yellow lights, pot holes marked by striped barriers and steaming tubes, one-way streets and no parking signs, pedestrians and commuter buses. Each obstacle took me to the next level, further from Shade, from Brooklyn, or wherever it was the game had begun this morning.

I was moving steadily ahead until I turned the wrong way down a one-way street. I dodged a few cars, my hands gripped tightly to the steering wheel. Vehicles honked in symphonic streams; then, an aria of screeches and obscenities. My pulse raced and I thought, I'm fucked. I heard myself scream. A UPS truck cut in front of me. I jerked the wheel to the left and skid to a halt, just missing a parked car. I shut off the ignition, took deep breaths as the quaking in my body subsided.

Seconds later, I looked up and saw I was across the street from a parking garage, it's neon sign flashing *deus ex machina:* Over here, stupid! I turned on the ignition and bolted across the street as if I'd known where I was going all along. When I stepped from my jeep, the garage attendants clapped and cheered. I suppose they were honored I'd taken on New York City traffic to make it to their garage.

From there, it was only a few blocks to the address Alexis had given me. I rode the elevator to the thirty-third floor and was directed down a carpeted hallway, quiet but for the clackety-clack of a few keyboards, voices murmuring room to room. I heard Alexis talking as I entered the edit suite, and though the heat pumped proudly throughout the facility, her voice chilled me more than the streets outside. "Well, well, my demon writer has arrived," she said, then turned back to the young man she'd been talking to. "Look, just get the Bran Flake people out of here, okay? They're driving me crazy, I mean, what do they make, like a thousand dollars a minute?"

"Something like that."

"And they're in here all night drooling over my low-budget pussy. Call the ad agency if you have to, just get them out." The man backed up a few feet and landed at the crowded edit bay. Alexis pointed her neck to the door, a gesture that soon had us entering the empty suite across the hall. She sat down in a black leather chair with wheels. I stayed standing. "They say the pen is mightier than the sword, but what about the evil tongue?"

"Am I fired or not?" I said, in no mood today for her perverted voir dire.

"I was ready to cut you a break after the scene with Wanda, but using my name like that." She swiveled in her chair, looked up at me. "Jesus, Rachel, the one thing I expected was a little discretion, that's the whole point."

"I know, I slipped up."

"Oh, you bet, and your slip is really showing this time. You're like a teenage boy who can't get laid."

Her words hit too close to home, made my cheeks flush with shame. Again, my heavy coat had me sweating as if I were in a sauna. Alexis shook her head. "My last ghostwriter used to buy me stuffed animals and tea, I have boxes and boxes back in the office; the one before that did novenas before she came on the set, they all seemed normal at first, too. You know, other people have problems with secretaries, me, I can't keep a ghostwriter."

"You don't want a ghostwriter. We always talked about me when I'm supposed to be writing your life."

"It's funny you say that, I haven't seen a word from you."

I sighed, leaned my hip against a steel console. It was true, I hadn't written a word. Even worse, I could no longer remember writing at all, nor what my life had been like with a day job. I'd phoned people, visited them, typed little stories into my computer. For this my paycheck passed directly into my checking account.

The biweekly checks had since diminished into strike pay, a pittance almost wrested from me by the union after the Gerri Michner incident. The union now had me on probation: One false move and into the poor house I hobbled. Faster, too, without the five-thousand-dollar advance Alexis had promised but as yet not tendered my way. I'd maxed out a couple of credit cards counting on that money. I needed the money.

So I did what any mildly self-respecting woman on the brink of losing her second job in four months would do: I groveled. Alexis listened, then wheeled sideways in her chair. "I'm sorry, but it's over," she said. My heart dropped to my stomach. I felt manipulated, as if she'd promised me stardom without telling me what I would have to do for it; how she would bring me to my knees, like a good little porn star begging for the money shot...*oh, baby, please come all over my face!*

Alexis stood, smoothed down her wool pants with painted fingernails. At that moment I would have sworn she was a man. Ultra-femme like Tricky in drag, but a man nonetheless, passing with the swish of her trousers and a whiff of herbal shampoo. In the dim hallway, she turned around. "I don't understand, I try to teach you young people what I know and it always backfires."

"Maybe you're trying too hard."

"I hope you get what you want, Rachel."

She returned to the edit suite, and I knew I would someday remember our parting as pivotal. What I hated was that Alexis knew it, too.

My apartment felt lonelier than ever. The message light blinked three, but I couldn't bear so much as listening to Shade...or Aunt Lorraine...or any human being. On the way home I'd vowed to abstain from human concerns, be they of the flesh or the spirit.

Instead, I grazed through my beleaguered check book, charting the stack of bills I'd before so happily ignored. Beneath my desk, Freddy circled, shoved her nose up against my shin. "You think you're hungry now, just wait," I told her, imagining the two of us fighting over the last tin of Fancy Feast.

I remembered Aunt Lorraine saying she'd left a little money for me, but I would have to kill her first and, although that was in fact what she'd requested, nobody would believe me if the sum were too large. There might be a courtroom scene like the kind I used to write about, then the headlines and column inches:

REPORTER ON STRIKE KILLS AUNT

> *Brooklyn, New York—Rachel Silver, a midlevel reporter at* The City News *before the Newspaper Guild went on strike last fall, was arraigned in State Supreme Court this morning after administering the suicide of her aunt, Lorraine Slivowitz. Although the family had been consulting with Milford P. Kaminsky, it is unclear whether the Master of Self-Deliverance was present at the time of death....*

Freddy mewed a few times before scratching hard at my knee cap. "Stop it or I'll call the ASPCA and have them put you to sleep!"

She backed away, and I felt awful, threatening her with euthanasia. I was so guilty I fed her an entire can of fishy wet food, and a bowl of crunchies. I watched her speckled stomach expand, her teeth clinking in kitty ecstasy against the glass bowl. She was too damn easy to please.

Back at my desk, I dug up the Ziploc bag of microcassette tapes containing the Alexis Calyx sessions. I hadn't transcribed one of them, perhaps knowing all along what I would find: that though I'd accepted the responsibility of deconstructing her life, it was she who'd done the deconstruction job on me.

> *Silver was recently fired from her second job as ghostwriter for Alexis Calyx, the erstwhile X -rated film star who has since become a producer of adult films herself. "I should have known better," Calyx said. "It's always those frigid types you have to worry about. . . ."*

I dropped the bag of microcassettes to the floor and jumped on top of it, crushing the plastic with my platform boots, smashing the tapes beyond use. My apartment suddenly stifling, I ripped off my sweater and threw it to the ground. It landed next to the pile of videotapes Alexis had given me, all of those fucking porno films. I stepped up to them, hoisted my leg back, and kicked the pile with full force, kicking and kicking until the videos covered the floor and I felt queasy for ever taking pleasure in them. Like a bulimic perusing her half-eaten packages of potato chips, pretzels, organic wheat sticks, fat-free Devil Dogs, her empty Dominos boxes, I needed to purge.

Into the kitchen I marched and grabbed the sharpest of my non-sharpening butcher knives. I took an old Alexis Calyx tape and forced the knife into its rigid white holes, the vagina dentata, stabbing until the black plastic cracked and the shiny brown tape came rolling out. I punctured another tape, watching on the wall the chiaroscuro of my arm rising and falling with the knife, and thinking myself a murderer. My limbs were buried in endless curls of videotape: dead movies. But I kept up the slaughter, finding my way toward *X-posure,* the movie that had so inextricably bonded me to Shade.

> *Silver, too, was involved in a lesbian love triangle with fellow News reporter Teesha Marie Simpson and biker chick Tina—*

who was a bitch, a motherfucker, a cunt; I hated her!

This stuff of supermarket tabloids set off my rubber band ball. I slammed the knife into the video and didn't stop until I was surrounded by plastic fragments like pieces of glass from a smashed window after a car wreck. The few nicks in my skin throbbed, but it still wasn't enough.

I opened my underwear drawer and removed the pop-gun, its pathetic cork flaccid, dangling. I snipped the string and the cork bounced to the floor. Into my mind floated the beginning of every Hebrew prayer I'd tried to forget: *Baruch atah adonoi*...pressure walled behind my eyes. I cut into the wood, determined to saw the whole thing off with a nonsharpening knife, a process that became as cumbersome as felling a Redwood. I found a hammer and banged until the shaft weakened into thin splints. I broke off each one individually. Nothing was left of the toy but its yellow handle. A half moon in my trembling palm.

The telephone rang. I plucked a few splinters from my fingers waiting on the message that eventually ushered in RR's voice. Always, a third party waiting in the wings, always another triangle. I picked up as he was about to sign off. "What do you want?"

"Fine, thanks, and yourself?"

"Alexis fired me," I said, video refuse collecting at my feet as I trudged in circles.

"Like everyone in New York didn't see that coming. You're too much like her."

"She said the same thing a few weeks ago, I just don't see it."

"The question is: are you a good bitch or a bad bitch?"

"I'm hanging up."

"Okay, I'll be right there."

"Where?"

"Your apartment."

"What are you talking about? I don't want to see you, I don't even like you."

"That's not important. We can go someplace, have a little fun."

I stopped pacing, sat down on the floor. "You want to have fun?"

"Yeah."

"With me?"

"Yeah."

"What makes you think I'm any fun? Do I seem like a fun-loving person?"

He laughed so I laughed, as relieved by the banter as I'd been earlier, happening upon that strategically placed parking garage. But my apartment was a mess, the kind of burglarized chic that followed a search for top-secret documents in spy movies: drawers hanging open, mountains of loose videotape, shards of black plastic everywhere, not to mention the wood shavings from my castrated pop-gun. No way was he coming over here.

"All right, I'll meet you downstairs."

"Just don't forget your toothbrush," he said.

Hanging up, I found myself lying on a bed of videotape. As if it were a religious ceremony, I collected a few pieces of tape in my fists and hurled them at the ceiling, laughing maniacally as the room drizzled with celluloid.

The films were mere training videos. I could be more Silver Ray than Rachel Silver, I even had the porn star's shaved pussy. Alexis had seen the transformation brewing; Shade, though intrigued, had tried to run from it; but RR all along had been waiting for this very moment.

I got up, went into the bathroom, and opened my medicine chest. Beneath the shelves, rust blistered into trails of desiccated tears. I removed my toothbrush, its splayed bristles reminding me of Shade, the week we'd shared just about everything in this apartment. My eyes oceaned over, and I knew I had to toss it. Silver Ray needed her own toothbrush.

Oh, Little Playmate

It was 2:10 a.m. in New York, 11:10 p.m. in Las Vegas when I gave up time. I was groggy-eyed and claustrophobic; ready to disembark at McCarran Airport. From the runway, I could see the cityscape glimmering like the rhinestones on one of Aunt Lorraine's sweatshirts. I thought of her lying in bed at home, that smell of her room that drove Mom crazy. Dying stinks like an airplane bathroom.

I wanted to turn around. Forgo the distant lights that kindled my amusement-park anxiety: the heart palpitations and head-spins, the sensory overload. My father once had a union buddy who worked the gate at Coney Island and gave us free tickets for the rides. I was very young the few times we went. What I remembered was Neil following me around the arcade and unbuckling our safety bar on the Cyclone. Now, Neil happened to be living somewhere inside those hills of screaming neon. I was already biased against this city.

RR yanked my garment bag from the compartment above us and turned to me. "Give me your watch," he said.

"What?"

"You're in my time zone now."

"I'll set it back."

"Un-uh," he nodded, making a curling motion with his forefinger. "Give it here."

In his eyes I saw the two of us together in the first-class bathroom just a few hours ago, the lens out of focus, but the stench of urine still so overwhelming I felt dizzy. Wanting only to get off the plane, I unsnapped the clasp of my watch and handed it over. His cheeks dimpled as if my relinquishing that little bit of control had contented him. I was on his time, in his world. As bullied as I felt, I pretended it was nothing, smiling as we left the airport, the way Silver Ray would do it.

The night was cold, yet nothing like the deep freeze we'd left back in New York. RR hailed a red and white taxi, and we climbed inside. For a quick second I was actually relieved not to have to make any decisions. To have everything taken care of.

"MGM," RR said.

"Huh?"

"Over there," he pointed to a glowing green microcosm that usurped at least five boulevard blocks. "Dorothy's inside...and Toto too."

"I thought she went back to Kansas."

"Yeah, but she couldn't find work. They all turn up here when the work stops."

"I hated that movie," I said. We were stopped at a traffic light, overshadowed by the sparkle of the emerald city. It was guarded by two irate-looking lions: wash-ups. Long past courage, anger was all they had left.

"Okay, next," he laughed, then pointed to the Tropicana. I started to relax, as we cruised the strip, a looking glass in motion with the windows rolled up and radio playing loud. Songs from boot-in-your ear country to neurotic rock fell in synch with the flashes of green of white of glittering gold; the exhaust of a million vehicles cast a filmy screen over the Day-Glo boulevard. Color dripped from the buildings, streamed like cars through time-lapse photographs. Everywhere, an assault of lights taking me back to the airplane cabin and its dingy stars, the noxious buzz of the airplane bathroom, where I'd let him in and kissed him like a porn star should. It just seemed the thing to do. For kissing him was easier than talking to him, though I couldn't help but notice how tight he kept his mouth, as if he couldn't stop sneering. I'd gotten used to Shade's lush and lulling lips, the way she tickled my gums with her tongue. My longing for her turned to anger. I tore open the buttons on RR's shirt and dug my fingernails into his chest as hard as I could. He pushed me up against the sink, lifting my shirt, biting down hard on my nipples. Violently he came to me, as if he were some kind of sexualized cyborg, a sci-fi version of Long Dong Silver. But he did have his human side, the one now reaching for my hand in the back of this cab reeking of pine antiseptic.

I held his hand, but kept my eyes glued to the window as we traversed the haphazard diorama of Western culture, slipping between medieval castles and circus clowns, the ancient pyramids, Paris, and New York, New York. Here, too, came Ronald McDonald dressed in a sequined tuxedo once owned by Liberace. It was a landscape that seemed familiar, as if the lights and the energy and the license had been neurologically implanted by three decades of television and movies. Just once I wanted to arrive in a place free of prefab imagery; I wanted to make it my own.

Still, the strip was bigger, louder, flashier than I had imagined. The town pumped like a massive strobe, with soap-box speakers cranking out the bass so the streets trembled. New York might have been the city that never slept, but Las Vegas never shut up. It pulsated with an aura of twenty-four hour foreplay, but no coming. Just like our mile-high expedition, the two of us, in the bathroom, fiddling endlessly with each other as if we were in combat, a residue of desperation clinging to the metal walls. Our pants had come down in synch. I traced the outline of his dick beneath his tight, thigh-length briefs. It was bigger than a breadbox, bigger than Barbie, much too big for me. A pang shot up my vagina. I fell backwards, and my head clapped against the mirror. Delirious, I asked if he had a condom.

"Shit." He sighed, his hands dropped to his sides. "Shit."

He stared at me, his face blue-balled, pent-up, moody, and aggressive. I was almost guilty enough to blow him as an act of mercy, but felt queasy and couldn't breathe; as if together we'd drained the last drops of air from the bathroom. We zipped up, banging elbows we were squeezed so close, even first class leaving too little room for sex gone bad. Up in the clouds, I thought I could be Silver Ray. I was wrong.

I would have given up on her entirely had we not found our way to Caesar's Palace. From the moment we walked through the thick glass doors and were greeted by the computerized clink-bing-bing of the slot machines, the place screamed Silver Ray's name. No matter that the machines and tables were crammed with people so obviously American with their bottle-blond hair and fancy jogging suits, their male-pattern baldness and wrinkled chino pants, inside we were all Romans. And you know what they say about being in Rome: let pleasure reign supreme and anyone be king or queen. Providing you had the dough.

I could only imagine the number of paychecks, credit cards, second mortgages that paved these roads to Rome. Me, I was on the porn-star package; all expenses paid. I fought another flash of the plane, turning instead to the tranced-out tourists dipping into their plastic coin buckets and bowing before the quarter slots as if they'd hit Mecca. It was a religious thing as far as I could tell, you pull, you pray.

RR cashed a few bills, and we practiced pulling and praying until the doorbells started giving me a headache. "What next?" I said.

He lifted me up against a dollar slot machine, slipped his knees in between my legs, and kissed me under the blaring lights of the casino. I tried to shut my eyes, be in the romance, but felt accosted by the ringing, the shouting, the clink of quarters jiggling in their containers. The fantasy hadn't kicked in yet. I pulled my head back.

"Ever play baccarat?" he said.

"I've never played anything." Because of my father's OTB habit, I would have worn the same pair of sneakers through four years of high school if it hadn't been for Aunt Lorraine. She always saw to it that I was taken care of. The thought of her hit me harder this time; here, where the fun never stopped. I grabbed the back of RR's neck and kissed him to make everything else start melting away.

He lifted me from the slot machine, and on the way to the table explained the rules of baccarat. "All you need to do is remember the numbers."

"I'm a verbal person."

"Change your thinking," he said.

Sitting down, I noticed a sign that said twenty-five-dollar minimum and almost gagged. "This is the James Bond game, isn't it?"

"You know more than you think."

"The name is Rod. Robbie Rod."

"All right, if that's who you want." He set down two stacks of chips in front of me. "Are you ready to play?"

"Yes," I nodded. It was a dull game, but for its high-rolling stakes. We simply bet on who would come closest to the number nine. I didn't like the other players betting on my hand, it upped the pressure to win, and when I felt pressured my performance faltered. I finished a glass of champagne and ordered another.

"You should bet higher," RR said.

"But I'm losing."

"You worry too much, it's kind of endearing, but enough already."

"It's your money," I said, and he smiled. I put down a couple of chips and bet on the dealer. RR did the same. Not only was it his money, but now I had him following my bets. And he was supposed to know the game. My teeth chattered against the champagne glass as I sipped. The dealer drew an eight, beating everyone at the table. I won! The dealer slapped down the chips in front of us and screamed: "Winner!"

"I like that, could you say that again!" I shouted. The player next to me rolled his eyes. "What?"

"It's etiquette," RR nudged me. "You don't talk like that to the dealer."

I shrugged. "It was a joke."

"Just play."

Gamblers had no sense of humor. Dad used to come home with OTB tickets hanging out of his pockets and swear on his life he wasn't gambling. The more Mom jeered at him, the more sober his contention. He hadn't been near the place, how dare she even suggest it.

I finished another glass of champagne, and this time played three chips, with RR following my lead. I lost. Everyone at the table smiled. I felt as if the walls were screaming: Loser! I needed another drink, I needed more money. I wanted to win again.

Thankfully, RR pulled out another roll of chips. As if he were dripping with cash. Maybe he was. I had no idea where his money came from; apparently he hadn't seen a movie through in years.

What if it were his second mortgage I was running through? His vacation fund? He was going to kill me.

Yet the more scared and guilty I felt, the more liberal I became in my betting. I was convinced I could get it back, save his house, his car, his credit rating. With a stack of chips in front of me, I even went for the near-impossible tie. RR looked at me as if I were crazy. This was the all or nothing play. Just before the dealer flipped, he pushed out his pile of chips and tagged along again. Oh shit, I thought. My head spun like a slot machine.

I almost fell off my chair when the dealer and I both came up with seven. "Winner!" he shouted. I jumped up and down as our chips multiplied. RR in an uncharacteristic burst of passion grabbed me and hugged me. The bells in Caesar's Palace sung simultaneously. "I am never leaving this casino!" I shouted.

My streak held out a while longer; no more big wins, however. The hotel comped us bottles of champagne, a steak dinner, and a limo home in the hopes of keeping us under its roof until we started losing again. I would have obliged, but RR made us quit. I'm not sure whether this was instinctive or because he had time on his side. There were no clocks in the casino. No windows. Nothing to distinguish one hour from the next, morning from evening.

Outside, night flashed electric. Like degenerate dignitaries we stepped into the house limo and set out for the proverbial dark, desert highway. Watching the strip shrink behind us, I thought it was probably morning in New York, one day since I found Tina Macadam at Shade's apartment. It seemed like weeks ago when I kept to the facts, minutes when I let emotion seep through the cracks.

An attempt to banish Shade from my thoughts found me looking out the window, but the emptiness mimicked my heart. I leaned back against the spongy vinyl seat. RR's arm stirred behind me. "Tired?" he said.

"Wired, actually." I bounced back up, turned toward him. "So, how much did I make?" He smiled. "Come on, tell me, tell me."

"A couple thousand, after you cut the losses."

"Come on, really."

"We were playing hundred dollar chips."

"Jesus, you're serious!" All night long I'd had no idea of the stakes, the chips were like Monopoly money to me.

"Beginner's luck," he said. "I promise you, it won't last."

"What does?"

"Now you're talking." He pinched my cheek, then looked out his window.

We were deep into nothingness. I could see the outline of a few black mountains surrounded by heavy clouds, inky air; space so empty I thought it counterfeit as a casino theme. It occurred to me then that I'd given up not only my notions of time and money, but any claim to place as well. For all I knew, RR and the chauffeur had made a pact to drag me into Death Valley and rape me or kill me or rough me up and sell me into the sex industry. It was almost anti-climatic when we pulled into the gravel driveway of his house in Boulder City, not too far from the Hoover Dam. He said you could hear the water crashing sometimes if you listened closely.

Once inside, the track lighting revealed a split-level spaciousness and too much glass. One entire wall was made of sliding glass doors. The others, painted sparkling white, housed shadows of numerous large cactuses that sprung up from the carpet, a garden of spikes and shafts arranged in ithyphalic absurdity. Did he have any idea what his walls reflected? Or was it just me? My fear of the priapic in general, his world-famous piece in particular. I shifted my gaze from the wall to his furniture, which betrayed a penchant for clean slick surfaces and seemed more about function than comfort—a lot of leather and lacquer and chrome that reminded me of an upscale law firm. I'd never seen so much space with so little personality.

He led me upstairs to a monstrous room, empty but for a platform bed with black sheets, a black Formica bureau, and a giant-screen television attached to a rack of VCRs and audio equipment. In the corners were two stereo speakers, each about my height. It was a teenage fantasy room, only without the rock-and-roll posters or magazine clippings of supermodels. The one photograph on the bureau was a framed picture of RR himself, a bit younger, in a suit and tie, shaking the hand of George Bush, the presidential seal and American flag behind them.

He dropped my bag. The weight of it hitting the floor exhausted me. At the click of a remote music filled the room. Slow, melodious chanting that sounded like a troupe of monks I'd once heard in California. I sat down on the edge of the bed and felt my body sink into the deep swish of water. I burst out laughing. "You have a waterbed!"

"There's nothing more comfortable," he said. Then he kissed me, and though I'd wanted to shower and brush my teeth and could barely steady myself on the bed, I kissed him back. Maybe it was the lure of the oscillating waves, the dreamy reverence of the music, or the lights that dimmed at his fingertips, but the room as much as my presence there suddenly made sense. I submerged myself further into the bed, giving over willingly as RR undressed me.

He touched and probed and tongued as if it had been a while since he'd been this close to another human body, although I sensed him stirring as he came to the space where my pubes were beginning to bud again. "You're shaved?"

"Long story," I said, again feeling Shade's presence as much as I felt his.

"Wait a minute, did you do something for Alexis? Did she put you in a scene?"

"No."

"I'm serious, did she?" He gripped my arms tightly and sneered as if we were back in the smelly airplane bathroom.

"No, I swear." I curled my fists and pushed out against his hands, those beautifully manicured fingers I'd first noticed in the Korean restaurant, the night he drew Silver Ray out of her cloister into his dirty-blue *mise en scène.* His thumbs dug into my biceps, waves rippled beneath us. I conjured all the strength I had into my arms and pushed harder, grunting and sweating like a weightlifter until he let go, laughing. My entire body throbbed.

Still on top of me, still goading me, he sighed. "I really like pussy hair."

You asshole, I thought, but for some reason I smiled. I reeled him in by his belt loops, feeling the disparity of my skin against his jeans. "Take these off," I said.

"Not yet." He kissed me again, and it was fast and deliberate. I matched every shift of lip, tooth, and tongue so he'd feel it. Before

Shade I'd never liked kissing so much, now I couldn't get enough of it. My senses were on epileptic, and I was relieved that somebody else could do this to my body. Somebody so different from her.

I felt a finger slip up inside of me and cried out. "Settle down," he said.

"I hope you have a condom this time."

"You need a new line, Silver."

"As far as I'm concerned that's the only line, you're a porn star."

He propped himself up on top of me. "Apparently, so are you."

"You know what I mean."

"Are you always this impatient?" He pulled out his finger so quickly it stung and left me wallowing in its absence. Leaning over me, he yanked open a drawer next to the bed. It was literally filled with condoms and jellies and oils and lubricants. I wanted to burst out laughing again but thought better of it. This was his idea of foreplay, perhaps: showing me how well-prepared he was. Like a Boy Scout. Or the proud man shaking the hand of a president. It was sort of endearing. He removed a few condoms, some oils, a small container of Astroglide, and set everything down on the night table.

"There we go," he said, grabbing the tube of oil or lube and squeezing the sticky liquid over my breasts and stomach. The smell of rainwater and lemon made me want to sneeze. RR slid on top of me, and we plunged further into the water. I felt like a slippery squid, an eel, a star-fucking starfish. He clamped a hand over my mouth and spoke into my ear. "Are we having fun yet?"

Unable to speak, I nodded no.

He moved his lips from my ear to my mouth and kept his hand there when we kissed. A finger from his other hand slid inside me. I bit his lip. He growled; I tasted blood.

"So that's what you want? To play porn star." He added a finger, and the back of my neck tingled. I was sweating from my temples, terrified he might rip me to shreds before I got his cock in me, that is if I could ever get that cock in me. I squealed a few times at the pressure of his fingers, but the harder he pushed the more I craved. I kept opening for him, expanding. "Tell me, Silver," he said, and it was a voice I hadn't heard before, lower and more guttural. "Tell me how badly you want me to fuck your bald porn-star pussy."

Pain shot up my vagina, but I didn't want him to take his hand away. He shoved me against the headboard, practically suspending me in the air with the weight of his arm. Looking down I saw the top of his palm inside me and said, "Oh fuck!"

"That's right, baby, fuck." He twisted his hand and I felt a knife slice up my spine. I screamed, tried to steady myself against him but could only grab a few strands of his hair before falling forward. He caught me with his left hand and the two of us, miraculously, were sitting upright on a waterbed, with his hand buried in my vaginal canal. "Let's go, I want to hear you say it."

"Fuck you!" I shouted. Lost with his wrist against my clit, his fingers ballooning inside me. I thought I might pass out from the pain, took a few quick breaths, then felt dizzy. He grabbed my neck with his free hand, tilting my head backwards.

"Not you," he said. "Me. Fuck me."

"Fuck you!"

"Me!"

"You!"

"Bitch!" I was stunned silent. That last word reverberated in the tones of the ancient monks. Our eyes met. He started to pull his hand away. I grabbed it and pushed it further into me, remembering how bad it felt before when he'd yanked out only one finger.

"Oh, excuse me," he said. "Do you want me to fuck you?"

I nodded.

"Then say it, and say it so I really hear it."

"Fuck me," I said.

"Not good enough." He glared, and I liked his anger, his arrogance, the way his eyes shifted to slits, and I wanted him to fuck me hard and not stop fucking me until I felt trashier than he kept saying I was. This is where I belonged, where I could perform: Silver Ray with her porn-star ass in the air. So I spoke this time as nasty as I could. "Fuck me, RR. Fuck me like I'm your porn star."

"Don't mind if I do," he said, pushing me down and carefully moving his fist inside of me. And there was pain, not the pain that comes from a paper cut or broken bone, but more like electroshocking surges of energy, the flicker of a light burning low, alluvial glow slamming into the bottom of the goddamn Hoover Dam. Damn. Robbie Rod made me a star. He of the polluted talk and snarling lips...made me feel strong in the sexiest Silver Ray way, made me want to scream so loud that Shade would hear me back in New York and know I was with somebody else. And know it was good because it wasn't her, wasn't anything but Robbie Rod deep-cunting Silver Ray deep into the Nevada night with the cameras rolling and the soundtrack pounding on and on and on.

We woke up to daylight. Streams of sun filtered through metallic blinds, splattering a painful glow throughout the room. RR stepped out of bed, and the lake beneath me trembled. He was still in his jeans. I was naked and dehydrated. He walked around to my side of the bed and kissed my forehead. His lips were soothing. A palliative. But I was too shy to get up until he left the room to make breakfast.

Downstairs, he whipped together an omelet out of an egg substitute—same kind they used on the space shuttle—and prepackaged vegetables. His food tasted delicious, the coffee stood strong as it should, and I wondered whether he'd drugged me or if, truly, I was starting to believe I might stay a while, here in the light of the desert sun, staring out of his dining room windows into mountains like milky-brown chocolate.

We ate quickly, then lingered over coffee, laughing, teasing each other. We wore sunglasses inside. I felt his hands reach for me underneath the table, my head thrown back in the warmth of morning, my bare foot in his denim crotch.

"Do something for me," he said, and I said sure. He said he wanted to watch me come. I sighed, jerked my foot from his lap.

"You want to know why I didn't."

"No, I want you to."

"Well, I don't."

"What do you mean, don't?" He stared at me and I thought, here we go again. I was still sensitive about the Tina Macadam episode, not to mention the years I'd spent listening to little Einsteins theorize about why I was so bad in bed: cold-hearted mother, hot-blooded father; late bloomer, early riser; repressed homosexual, hard-pressed in general. It was my fear of commitment, my need for control, something I'd eaten, too much caffeine, whatever.

The way RR was staring I knew it was coming. "You don't at all?" he said.

"Not with people."

"What then, with animals?"

"Yeah, me and Catherine the Great." I pursed my lips. He looked perplexed. "She died fucking a horse."

"No, that was Queen Elizabeth."

"She's not dead yet, moron."

"I think you're wrong."

"And while we're on the subject, I don't remember you getting off. You're still wearing your pants!"

"What can I say, it's not what interests me."

"Oh, bullshit."

"Seriously," he nodded. "I'm leather dick. You can stroke me, scrape me, suck me, bang it up all you want, or kiss me gently, I'm totally resistant. Always have been."

"You don't come?"

"Of course I do, but at my discretion. I can hold out forever or shoot on command. You're forgetting who I am."

"A real prototype."

He laughed. "So you don't with other people, but you do alone, but what about by yourself with somebody watching?"

"That's sort of stupid."

"Okay, what if it wasn't stupid? What if, actually, there was a reason, a wager so to speak?"

"Go on." I felt the insides of my rib cage warm, like photosynthesis, as if I were conducting a superhero transformation from frigid female to porn star. He took out a huge wad of cash. Hundreds.

"Here's the deal," he said. "You start, you know..."

"To masturbate."

"Yes, thank you. Every sound you make, moaning, screaming,

whatever, I give you a hundred bucks, and then when you come...oh, I don't know, let's make it five hundred."

"Dollars? Five hundred dollars?"

"Not enough?"

"No, no, fine. But how do you know it's real?"

"I trust you."

I stretched the elastic band of my satin boxers, summoning Silver Ray. She'd gotten me through the long hours of the night, the scene that left the insides of my vagina raw. I was thankful he didn't want to fuck me this morning, but this seemed an odd substitute. "Wait a minute," I stopped myself. "How do I know I can trust you?"

"You've seen the money, everything I've got is out on the table."

"Everything?"

He put a hundred dollar bill in front of me. "Everything. Now, let's see your fingers."

"I thought you trusted me." I pulled down my boxers with my left hand so he could see me touching myself with the other. He smiled, and I knew I didn't trust him, but it had little to do with money. It was that somewhere back in New York he'd crept into my fantasies; somewhere between our first dinner and that day on the set with Wanda Lynne's boots, he'd sussed out my burgeoning romance with the sex industry. He could tell I wanted to play porn star, only not for the camera.

I let out an audible sigh. He dropped another hundred on the table. I tried to be in the moment, click on Silver Ray, but Shade stalked my memory. We were at the Tannon benefit, standing outside in the freezing cold: *You don't know what you want, Slivowitz. It's like we're all part of your big experiment.*

"Talk to me," RR said, bringing me back to the mountains of Boulder City. I looked at him, confounded by his own part, why he was so eager to indulge me. "How old were you when you first did this?"

"I don't know, nineteen, twenty."

"So late?" he said, adding a bill to the pile.

"It never occurred to me," I lied. I wouldn't set a finger to my body while Neil was still living at home. Once, I'd even gone a week without showering after he'd drilled the holes in the bathroom wall.

Another hundred hit the table, and I was as rebellious as a horse-fucker, here in Neil's city, but on my terms: Screw you big brother and the city you live in. I felt my cheeks flush, let out a sonorous oh. One more bill on the table. I looked at him, suddenly self-conscious. "I can't believe this."

"Sure you can, you just want me to tell you it's okay, you want my blessing. I'm like a priest."

"I'd prefer rabbi."

"Do rabbis hear confessions?"

"I don't care."

"Do they make you feel slutty for touching yourself? You feeling slutty, Silver?"

"Shut the fuck up," Silver Ray shouted.

"Yeah, that's it." He put down another bill. "I love it when you say fuck. You sound like a filthy debutante."

"Fuck."

"That for me?"

"All yours."

He smiled. The money pile multiplied, and we were back in the casino. Only it was his table, his rules. I was playing again, the stakes Silver-Ray high. I didn't want to lose. I would fake it rather than lose.

His words garbled; I was through with them entirely. Slipping in and out of real time. Through the window I caught the line of the burning sun. The shimmer of water. Me wearing sunglasses, double-exposed on the lenses of his sunglasses. On his face together: me and Silver Ray.

"Come for me, Silver," he said, and I thought, yes, I could, because it was tied to nothing but Monopoly money; yes, I would, because it was all an act anyway. There was no past, no future, no sweat, no strings, no goddamn desert shut-down. I could let it go, let myself slip from gibberish whispers to sweet, inescapable screams. I'm rich, I thought or might have shouted. So fucking rich! He started counting out loud: One-Two-Three...I screamed until my voice went hoarse, and I collapsed on top of the dining room table.

"Silver," he said. "You just made yourself twenty-one hundred dollars!"

"Blackjack." I could barely breathe.

He leaned across the table, lifted my cheeks in between his hands. "You're beautiful," he said.

I smiled, "Your turn, leather dick."

People have always accused me of being cheap. Personally, I view myself as more of a fiscal conservative; I don't take many vacations or eat in fancy restaurants, unless of course it's on someone else's tab, and until recently, I used to calculate my expenses to number of hours worked, a habit I'd picked up during my waitressing days in college. So it was no surprise that at the end of our masturbatory interlude I was still up thirteen hundred dollars.

But who cares about the money, I got his pants off. Then, upstairs, in the chalky light, I knelt down before him with a wooden ruler. (In my frenzy to leave New York it had somehow ended up in my bag.) He found this amusing. He said he'd never let anyone measure him before. He was erect. I held his penis against the ruler and its head hit the groove at two. He was only ten inches! And lean. Manageable, perhaps. I ran my fingertips up and down the silky shaft and my throat constricted. I wanted it inside me so badly, but wouldn't let him know. I took a deep breath and sat back on my ankles. "The camera adds a few pounds," he smiled, and two oval dimples chiseled into his unshaven cheeks. He had light purple rings underneath his eyes. He looked scruffy and attentive. I leaned over and kissed him.

The kiss dissolved into a forty-eight hour game of truth or dare as money changed hands and gels squirted into orifices and showers were taken and food was carted in from the family restaurant in town. When I finally got him inside me it was almost anti-climactic, not nearly as dramatic as all the begging he made me do for it. And to fuck a porn star was an expensive scenario. He gave it to me at a steal for five hundred bucks. I felt like a contestant on an X-rated game show. *I'd like to buy a blow job please....* Had he let me, I would have spent every last hundred watching him come. I loved how the moment made him tiny and beetlelike, reduced him to nothing but the stream of his semen. It was where he lived for me. But he had a similar vision. He paid absurd amounts of money to finger my asshole while I brought myself off, which I did with alarming ease. As if in those concupiscent hours I'd shed more than a few layers of skin.

Why he'd taken me into his bed, however, still puzzled me. Surely, he could have paid any number of women to play these games, and in his life there had been so many lovers, both on and off screen. Maybe I did remind him of Alexis. Or he had a thing for the orgasmically challenged. Or it was just something to do.

I worried he was getting bored. No way could this be enough, could I be enough. I kept waiting for him to snap out of his trance and ask, "Who are you?" A question I couldn't answer with the slightest bit of clarity, reduced as I was to a piece of pulsating flesh, one minute surfeited in ecstasy, the next choking back tears. But whenever he tickled the inside of my knee with his toe, scratched his fingers against my back, or told me I looked good naked, sailing casually upon the stained black sheets, I submitted hoggishly to the next round. It took two days before my stomach constricted at his touch and I found myself stifling a yawn. Maybe *I* was the one getting bored.

He climbed on top of me. "Should we go somewhere tonight?"

My resounding yes came too quickly, but I felt almost as claustrophobic as we'd been in that airplane bathroom. I wanted to get out of the house and be public. We needed a few supporting characters. That was the difference with Shade, I never wanted to be anywhere else.

He got up out of bed and cranked the lights a little, giving a cocktail lounge effect. The music reminded me of crooners in polyester. RR, my celluloid hero, this man with the invincible penis, was mad about barber shop quartets. It made me want to pinch his cheeks. Then I felt guilty for wanting to leave the bedroom. "Where to then?" He stood half-cocked, his hair puffed up like a seaman's cap. "Caesar's? Downtown?"

"Let's go to a different place, somewhere sleazy."

"Sleazy," he nodded, clicking his tongue against the roof of his mouth as he lumbered into the bathroom. He must have liked the idea.

Downstairs, dusk had sucked its way through the water and up into the well-carved mountains. By the time we got to Vegas night had fallen, and the desert, rugged and timeless by day, was obliterated in a multiple birth of neon.

We ate dinner at a Japanese restaurant, played a few rounds of blackjack, before RR took me to a place called The Rocking Horse. It was down-scale and exactly what I'd imagined a Vegas strip bar to be. A smoke-filled laziness was the lay of the land, offering stark contrast to the pump of fresh oxygen that jolted the casinos. Atmospheric pressure here rendered itself in visuals.

We drank flat beer. RR watched me watching the women dance in front of us. My favorites were the theme dancers: the Wall Street banker, the cowgirl, the Wal-Mart cashier. I found their artifice comforting, for these women were no more executives and shopkeepers and schoolgirls than I was Silver Ray. We were all traveling through the land of make-believe, paper moons and canvas skies as far as the eyes could see. Even naked, the veneer never faltered. Yet their writhing bodies gave voice to my longing. How much I missed seeing naked women, one naked woman really.

Then, as if on cue, came a vision in white taffeta over lustrous cocoa-brown limbs, her hair braided and beaded just like Shade's. She shimmied up to us under a sexed-up syncopation, a gloriole of spots and smoke rings, saintly in her transparent gown, and a resemblance so strong I had to fight the desire to jump up on stage with her. Did this make me sexist? Misogynist? I didn't give a damn, with the way she swung her legs around the silver pole at the end of the bar, pirouetting like a championship figure skater, before she was back in front of us, on her knees in a slow, rhythmic grind.

I followed her back and forth, watching as she discarded her billowing robe, teased the straps of her bleach-white lingerie in her own dance of the seven veils, and if I'd become Herod to her Salomé, so be it. It was my head she was dancing for.

"We can buy her if you want," RR said, but I shushed him away, pretended he was just another annoying interloper. Besides, I was sick of all the buying and selling. I wanted to give the rest of my money to Salomé and be poor again.

Salomé flung off her bra and was left in her garter, g-string, and white pumps. What talent set against the dreariness of the club. I reached into my pocket and took out a hundred dollar bill, thinking this had to be one of the craziest things I'd ever done. I rolled the bill tightly, waved my hand in the air, reeling with its power, its privilege. She came to me, bent at the knees, and I started to sweat. Fingers shaking, I stuffed the bill in her garter, unable to look at her.

"Wow! Thanks a lot," she said, and her voice sounded as if she'd just inhaled a balloon full of helium. With those few words, the entire picture burst.

Salomé left the stage, Ben Franklin in tow, for a trip down lap-dance lane with some slovenly drunk. I eyed her for a little while, until I must have looked as bored as the rest of the men sitting beneath the cavalry of women in fancy pajamas.

"How does it feel?" RR chided me.

"You think it's funny. So I gave a hundred dollars to a woman who sounds like Mickey Mouse."

"She deserved it. You should have seen your face while she was dancing."

"I wish she hadn't said anything though." I stood up and gave him a tug around his neck. "I'm going to the bathroom."

The door had a big sign that said, "Girls Only." I peed and went to the row of sinks where two dancers were preening. A slow night, they agreed, one helping the other find an unmarked patch of stocking to catch the snaps of her garter. Slow night? They hadn't met the grasshopper from New York yet.

I bummed a cigarette from the bestockinged brunette, sympathized with her about the scarcity of stockings because everyone nowadays wore panty hose. "What's a slow night?" I asked.

"Depends," the other one, an older-looking redhead, said. "What do you do?"

"Actually, I'm unemployed."

"Well, girlfriend, why didn't you say so?" the brunette said, jumping down from the sink, yanking up her stockings. In a flash I had the rundown: no total nudity, free drinks, dances anywhere from five to ten minutes, lap dances negotiable, make anywhere from a few hundred to a thousand bucks a shift. "Nothing compared to the scene on the strip," both women lamented, as if too many nights at The Rocking Horse had already squelched their dreams of rising through the ranks. As they spoke I couldn't stop thinking about the cash I'd been making on my orgasms; how I'd given up for money what I'd never been able to do for love. The money wasn't even real to me, as if it were worthless outside city limits.

Before leaving the bathroom, I took out my wad and handed each of the dancers one hundred dollars. "What are you, nuts?" the brunette said. The redhead raised her eyebrows, gritted her teeth at her friend.

"I'm with a guy outside, dance on his lap or something."

"Together?"

"Sure, why not?"

I left the bathroom and found RR. We walked to a darker bar in the back, where I became more interested in the men watching the dancers than the dancers themselves. Disengaged, emotionless, the men mirrored the lackluster zombies who sat at the slot machines all night long. No wonder they kept the sex separate from the gambling. Too much of the undead at play was enough to depress anyone.

My gaze fell upon the empty, black walls and swung a while with the flickering light of the disco ball. I turned my head to the left and caught a fleeting murmur of familiarity. As if I were reacting to an image in a dream, I thought, Oh, no, Neil's here. Slammed with a heavy techno beat, streaks of light, I blinked my eyes. This happens often: You're in a place where you know someone else is, and you see that person on the faces of strangers. I stepped forward to get a better look. Stared down the pudgy face that could have been Neil's, although I remembered him as being much thinner. He returned my stare, and even in the haze I could see those eyes so much like my own, that nose, Dad's could-have-been-a-movie-star nose, if only the rest of the package had come through as well.

The last time I'd seen Neil was at Grandpa's funeral, when he almost knocked over the casket fighting with Mom before the service. He was so obviously high, he couldn't stay seated. I think that was the day he hit Grandma.

A heavy-metal clanking, words like prayer, kill, and slaughter backing up a dancer with leather chaps and pierced nipples, as Neil and I moved toward each other. Part of me wanted to kick him in the balls for the hell he'd put me through as a child, but I also felt sorry for him. Finding him here, I knew he hadn't changed much. Me being here, now that was something to write home about.

He stood in front of me, balder than I'd remembered, with a gold chain hanging from his neck.

"Is Ma dead yet?" he said.

"Far from it, she's getting married."

"Oh." He nodded his head up and down as if something made sense. "This a friend of yours?" he said, pointing his head toward RR who'd come up behind me. "You a private dick or the real thing?"

"Who's this jerk?" RR said.

I took a deep breath. "He's my brother."

"Brother? I didn't know you had a brother."

"I've got two, actually."

"Listen," Neil said, a large vein pulsating in his keg of a neck. "I think I know who you are, and I don't owe them shit back on the Coast. Ask anyone, it was all a set up."

"He lives here? Why didn't you tell me you had a brother here?"

"I don't know, it never came up," I said, realizing then that I didn't want RR to know I had a brother, a mother, that I'd once had a father, too. Being with him was about being brand spanking new, like his furniture.

"You should have told me," RR said.

"Why?"

"Because you should have."

Neil slammed his hand on the bar causing RR and me to jump back a few steps. "All right, what the fuck is going on!" Neil screamed. "I want to know what you're doing here, Rachel. If he's not a cop, who sent you?"

I was about to answer when the two dancers from the bathroom joined us, and for some reason assumed Neil was the guy I'd wanted them to work over. They started hanging on him, calling him baby. His face reddened and on instinct I backed up. "Get the hell away from me!" he screamed.

"It's okay, honey, she already paid," the redhead said.

"Who?"

She pointed to me. Neil's eyes flared. He swung his arm out in front of him, shoving off both the redhead and the brunette. The redhead fell back against the wall and hit her head. I wanted to drop to my knees and beg her forgiveness. It was all my fault, trying to buy her with RR's money. I started moving toward her, but Neil stopped me.

"Get back!" he said.

RR pushed past my shoulder and, as if in time-delay, I saw him swing back his arm and crack his fist across Neil's face. Neil tripped backwards. I was stunned, as if he'd hit me, too. I remembered Neil as being invincible. A part of me wanted to throw my arms around RR, but I sensed that was the last thing I should do. He looked even angrier than Neil did.

Within seconds, a couple of goons in black flight jackets were escorting the three of us out the front doors into a hostile torrent of sunlight. I hadn't realized we'd been out that long. Neil rubbed his cheek and spit out a wad of blood.

"All right, let's go, Bozo," RR said.

"I want to talk to my sister."

"What makes you think she wants to talk to you?"

"Leave us a minute." I grabbed RR's wrist, not knowing what I was I trying to do. I was so out of my league and in the goddamn daylight. This must be what hell is, neon and brimstone in the morning. My brother's face in the light of dawn.

Thankfully, RR walked back to his Pathfinder. "All right," Neil said. "What are you doing in Vegas, what are you doing *here?*"

"I'm on vacation."

"At The Rocking Horse?"

I shrugged. "Yeah, I don't know what else to say."

"Why didn't you tell me you were coming?"

"No, you don't understand. I wasn't planning on seeing you."

"I don't trust you, Rachel. Something's up." Neil reached into the front pocket of his jeans and took out his wallet. He handed me a business card. I quickly read the bold letters: Neil DeSilva, Betting Consultant.

"You're still Italian?"

Neil winced. "You come by if you want, but leave your boyfriend home." He touched his cheek again. "I owe that guy one."

"Forget it, okay."

He nodded reluctantly, and we said goodbye. I knew he was watching me walk back to the Pathfinder and climb inside. But RR wouldn't move, let alone start the car. We sat silently waiting for Neil to leave the parking lot in his bright orange pickup truck. "What's that?" RR pointed to my hands.

"His card."

RR ripped it from my fingers. "A betting consultant," he laughed. "Scumbag." He dangled Neil's card in front of me, but when I reached for it, he pulled it away. We played this hand a few more times.

"Come on, give it to me!"

"What'll you do for it?"

I rolled my eyes, pleaded. He turned up his lip and pretended to tear the card. "Don't!" I said. He smiled his fuck-you smile, and I knew I was defeated. "What do you want?"

His right hand pushing my head into his lap said it all. The smell of stale beer and ashtrays clung to his jeans. I unzipped him, hoping to rip out a few pubic hairs, but found him protected by his briefs. He was already hard when I squeezed my lips around him. "You think you're so smart," he said. "That you're just playing." I tried to break free, but the harder I tried, the harder he gripped my hair. I wanted to slice my teeth through his ten or twelve inches; what difference did it make, I still gagged. But I was afraid of hurting him so badly he'd hurt me even worse. His shoulders jerked forward and his breathing grew heavier.

"Look at yourself, Silver." He pushed deeper into my throat. "Sucking cock in the parking lot of a titty bar."

All I could think was I had to make him come, swallow him down, but I knew he was holding out for the finish, the proof on Silver Ray's featured face. I cupped both of my hands around the base of his cock to keep from suffocating. His thrusts came faster, slapping against the back of my throat. I felt mucus dripping from my nose and wanted to vomit. Instead, I pushed both of my hands against his thighs and sprung up, heaving. He aimed, I shifted forward, and he hit the side of my neck, my hair, the collar of the jean jacket I'd borrowed from him. Not my face.

I wiped my neck with the sleeve of his jacket. He zipped up his pants, reached into his back pocket and handed me Neil's card. I took it, disgusted with myself. Worse than doing it for money, this had been about my brother. "We can go now?" he said, tentatively, as if I'd been the one begging for it and he'd simply complied. "Well?"

"Yes."

He started the engine and backed out of the parking lot. The strip, languid in the morning light, sagged behind us as if someone had pulled the life support on the entire city. I leaned my elbow against the window and stared out into the burnt bric-a-brac mountains, counting the Joshua trees all the way home.

The Thirty-Foot Cowboy

RR stopped the Pathfinder in front of the address on Neil's business card. Though he said he wasn't happy about me visiting Neil, he sensed he couldn't keep me locked away in his desert tower all day long. "How about one for the road?" he said. "We can do it right in front of his house."

His anger from the parking lot returned, and after he'd been sort of sweet yesterday, letting me sleep a while, then cooking salmon for dinner. We ate by candlelight, watched a couple of John Wayne movies. Daybreak found me alone on the leather couch with a comforter draped over my fully clothed body. I was glad to be by myself, but couldn't help feeling insecure. I got lost in that house without his hands on me.

"That was a joke," he said.

"I'm laughing inside." I jumped out and slammed the door behind me. The day was too perfect, hot enough not to need a jacket, with a light wind blowing. RR rolled down his window, stared; I wished for rain.

"What?" I balanced myself on the curb. He kept looking, as if he wanted to say something but couldn't get it out. "What?"

"Nothing."

"Then go already. I can make it to the front door on my own."

"Just remember, I know his phone number." He fired the ignition. I watched the Pathfinder drift down the road, sandwiched between identical rows of stucco houses with waffled orange roofs. I took a deep breath and sat down on the curb until ten cars passed.

When I was confident he'd gone, I walked a couple of blocks to a busier intersection and called Shade from a payphone. I needed to hear her voice, needed to know she was still there. Her machine picked up. I felt my lips tremble and started rambling, words about it being too early, or too late. "Are you there?" I screamed. "Yes? No? Maybe? Shit!" I slammed down the phone, but held onto the receiver with both hands as if I were choking it. My head fell against the back of my hands. I shut my eyes and listened to the cars streaming by, the rap of jackhammers across the street. I was so alone.

Walking back to Neil's, I passed the rows of houses like condos at a vacation resort, some with American flags hanging out front the way I remembered the stoops of Bay Ridge on patriotic holidays. But it was just another day in sprawling Las Vegas, where every day was the Fourth of July. It was still morning in America out here.

Neil's house did not have a flag out front. Instead there were a few spiky flowers hanging from macramé planters, and in front of the door was a fuzzy mat that said "Welcome." I thought of the sign Neil had plastered on the basement door when he'd moved down there—"Keep out: I break wrists."

A boy wearing baggy clothes and a baseball hat turned backwards met me at the door. I asked for Neil and he pushed open the screen door, motioning for me to enter with the flick of his neck. I loathed teenagers, the way they thought they owned the universe with their untied sneakers, their feckless aplomb. As we stepped inside to the smell of cigarettes and dog hair, he screamed, "Yo Ne-al!" No answer. He screamed again, this time hopping up the staircase to the left of the foyer. "Ne-al! There's a lady here!"

Lady? I saw myself more as the kid's contemporary than Neil's, or RR's for that matter. Alexis had called me on my latent spurt of adolescence, the raging hormones and braggadocio outside, while inside crept that forever-awkward, I'm-never-gonna-get-laid feeling. It hit me big here in Neil's living room.

Magazines were strewn about the floor: *Rifle Enthusiast, Vegas Week, Modern Gaming.* There were newspapers opened to the point spreads with numbers circled; there were teen boy things, a baseball bat, hockey skates, stacks of video game cartridges; there were also shotguns, a double barrel lying out on the coffee table, and a couple more on the shelf above a torn easy chair.

Footsteps and muffled voices coming downstairs shook me. Get this over with quickly, I thought. Neil appeared, followed by the boy, and I realized I was touching the shotgun on the table.

"It ain't loaded," Neil said. "No bullets allowed in the house."

"Oh." I pushed the gun away.

Neil nodded. "Want a beer?"

"Do you have anything without alcohol?"

"Right," he squinted at the boy. "Sonic, get my sister here a...Coke, okay? Good, go on and bring me one, too."

Neil settled back into the easy chair, flinging his battered cowboy boots in the air. "In case you were wondering that's his real name."

"Oh."

"He was born on the airforce base, so she named him Sonic. Better than 747, right?" I laughed, though I wasn't sure it had been a joke. Neil explained that "she" was Vera Dooley, his girlfriend, and this was her house. He'd moved in a few years ago. They weren't married, but they were a family, at least more of a family than we'd ever been back in Brooklyn, he assured me. His words brought the same smothering spitefulness I felt whenever Mom and Hy discussed their wedding plans, as if they had one up on me in the game of life, underscoring my own losing streak.

I was surprised by how much Neil with his run-on sentences reminded me of Mom. He talked nonstop until Sonic returned with our Cokes. "She don't look like your sister," he said.

"What's that mean, shithead?" Neil said and the familiarity of his tone chilled me. "Nothing." Sonic dropped his droopy teenage shoulders, looking lankier than before, almost shy even. "It's just that she looks kind of normal."

"Hah, hah...you're so fucking funny."

"No, really, she's the nine."

"Thanks," I said. It wasn't his language, but the way his eyes lit up that told me being the nine was a good thing. Like in baccarat. I looked down at my feet and thought it was the jeans and platform boots that nined me. Still, the kid wasn't so bad.

"All right, you're interrupting a private family moment," Neil said. "Get out of here, go practice shoplifting or something."

"Shut up!" the boy shouted. His cheeks and neck clouded pink.

I felt badly and wanted to defend him. Being with Neil always forced me to take sides.

Sonic grabbed his skateboard from the floor with a quick swish. "What's the matter, you embarrassed?" Neil cackled. "You should've thought about that before you forgot to clip the magnet bars; you steal like a spic."

The kid backed away, leaving the screen door bouncing behind him. I was suddenly afraid of him being gone, of being left alone with my brother, who was laughing so hard I could see the brown stains on his teeth.

"Little shit," he muttered, and I felt three decades of anger starting to brew. Neil tilted his head back and sipped from his Coke bottle. I tried to pretend we were just beginning, popping up in cement like the blocks outside. What would I say if we had no history, if we hadn't shared anything but a couple of Cokes on a sunny afternoon?

"This must be a nice place to live," I said.

"The weather's okay, at least in winter."

"Yeah, it's kind of like Miami in the day and New York at night." I took a swig of soda, felt the bubbles choke the back of my throat.

"So, you ready to tell me why you're here?"

I took a deep breath. "It's just what I said, I'm on vacation. I had to get away, I mean, things kind of suck at home, you know...with Aunt Lorraine."

"What about her?"

"Nobody told you?"

He shrugged and held open his palms. "What?"

"She's got cancer," I said, stopping to catch my breath. I hated saying it out loud: every time. I managed to keep my emotions in check as I continued, telling Neil about Mom and her Norma Desmond dramatics, Rowdy and his video camera, Kaminsky and his suicide pamphlets. But I left out the promise I'd made to Aunt Lorraine. Whether I went through with it or not, it would remain between the two of us.

Neil asked no questions, letting me talk until I couldn't think of anything else to say. After a brief silence, he rolled his eyes. "See, I knew something was up, I just felt it," he said. "It should have been

Mom." I stared at him, his blank smirk making me feel as if I were conspiring with the goddamn devil. I'd thought that myself, but never said it out loud. Somehow, Neil and I had ended up on opposite sides of the emotional spectrum: I felt guilty merely thinking certain things, while he seemed to act without consequence. He lit a cigarette and a craving enveloped my lungs, my throat.

"Give me one of those, would you?"

He threw me the pack, then a purple bic. "Didn't think you would smoke."

"I don't really." I lit a cigarette and inhaled deeply, staving off the jumpy feeling in my stomach, if only temporarily. Neil stared at me. I picked nervously at the white hairs on my jeans. "Do you have a dog?" I asked.

"A mastiff, or so she says. He's really a mangled German shepherd—Henry, king of the tool shed. The thing's older than Sonic, blind so he's got all this crap in his eyes and has to wear this plastic funnel around his neck. If I had my way I'd shoot him and get it over with."

"I know what you mean."

"Not Vera, she's into natural shit. She bathes him with Epsom salts and feeds him Metamucil. Got to keep him regular, says it's better for everyone this way."

I was about to ask who's everyone when I heard the screen door fly open and the sound of something hitting the floor. I turned my head. At the stairs a girl stood in leggings and a big T-shirt that made her look like a shrunken health club addict. She smiled at me, though the movement of her lips seemed tentative, sad. Her eyes, too, were a somber sort of brown, like my own.

"Dammit, Ivory! Get back here and help me!" called a voice from the doorway.

"You heard her," Neil said, and she scrambled away without looking at him.

The thought of my brother living with a prepubescent girl made me nauseous. All of the holes he'd drilled in the walls, the broken locks on my bedroom door, everything I tried to forget with a Coke and a smile came rushing back, and I remembered how much I'd once wanted to hurt him. I couldn't fight him off the way I'd learned to do with Rowdy, kicking him in the knee caps every time he smacked me or slammed a deck of cards over my knuckles until they bled. Neil never fought with his hands; not once did he touch me. He was more like an evil telescope, always watching, always knowing more than he should. I didn't know enough not to believe him when he told me my nipples were too small for my breasts or said the birthmark inside my right thigh made me deformed. Nor when he blamed me for Dad's death.

I'd been sitting at the kitchen table, studying for finals with a pile of cashew nuts and a large bottle of diet soda in front of me. I remember having to pee, but was holding it as long as I could. By the time I finally ran to the bathroom, I thought I would piss on the floor. The bathroom door only budged a few inches. I leaned up against it with all my weight, pushing and heaving until I fell through the doorway and landed on top of my father's body. He was crouched in front of the toilet, eyes wide open, pants down to his ankles. I jumped up and screamed. Then I peed in my pants.

Neil came running. "Poor bastard." He bent down, grabbed Dad's wrist and then looked up at me. "What were you doing in the bathroom with him?" he said.

Too shaken to say anything, I just cried.

"You probably killed him," he said and walked off, leaving me wailing on the bathroom floor with my dead father. At that moment, I knew Neil had no soul, and in the few years that followed my hatred of him became a physical thing. I nurtured it with fantasies of graduating from college and getting out of my house. But whenever my brother came within a few feet of me, I felt the twitch behind my left eye, a cramping in my neck and shoulders.

Those sensations flooded back, though Neil was a man I hardly knew, a man well into his thirties with rolls of fat around his stomach and hair loss settling in. Still, his every movement seemed aggressive, the way he kept crossing his legs and fiddling with the lever of the easy chair, how he twisted his gold pinky ring. He tapped into the worst of my violent impulses, made me feel as if I could actually harm somebody. No wonder they banned bullets from the house.

The movement of bodies slinking across the carpet told me I had to calm down. Vera Dooley appeared with the girl attached to her hand. "Well, hello there," Vera smiled. I said hello, but couldn't get beyond the scars on her face, like teardrops running down each cheek.

Vera sat down on the couch next to me with the girl clinging to her leg. She whispered something in her mother's ear. "It's Neil's sister," Vera said. "She came all the way from New York City where the World Trade Center is, don't you want to say hi?"

"No," she murmured through clenched lips, brought her feet up to the couch, and rested her elbows on her knees: pre-teen defiance.

"She's got a thing against talking," Neil said.

"That's not true," Vera said. "She's a little shy maybe; I was the same."

"Me too," I said. "How old is she?"

"Ivory, come on, tell her how old you are."

The girl looked over in my direction, staring fiercely, but didn't speak. She buried her head back in between her elbows. Vera, stroking her daughter's muddy brown hair, said, "She's ten. I know what you're going to say—she's small for her age. But she's big on brains. Right, honey?"

"Rocket scientist," Neil said.

"Look who's talking," Vera said. Her scars stretched and released, as if she were really crying. She couldn't have been much older than me, yet she had a weather-beaten look about her that made her seem generations away. Maybe it was the kids, or her clothes, the white running shoes and jogging suit of crinkled nylon like those Mom had taken to wearing these past years.

"So what brings you to Vegas?" she said.

"She's on vacation, with some dickhead boyfriend," Neil said.

"He's not my boyfriend."

"Oh, what a relief."

"Would you act human, please?" Vera said. "You want her going back and telling everyone what a jackass you are?"

"That's okay," I said. "We wouldn't want to change anything at this point."

Vera laughed. "You two got the same sense of humor."

I cringed at the thought of having anything the same as my brother. He cranked the lever on his easy chair, lit another cigarette.

"So what do you do back in New York?" Vera asked me.

"I'm a reporter, at least I was until we went on strike last fall."

"Oh that's right, I saw it on TV."

"What did it look like out here?"

"I don't know, like everything else, I guess."

"I saw a woman on TV from New York," came Ivory's muffled voice from between her knees. "She used to be a man and then she married a man who said he wanted to be a woman too. It was messed up."

"I'll say," Vera said. She kissed the top of her daughter's head. How light she seemed, so tender I'd almost forgotten the scars on her face. I had to know who'd cut her like that, if my brother was in some way responsible.

Neil smoked silently, eerily. Vera turned her attention back to me. "Listen, you're a writer and all...I got tons of stories, you should come and see me at the casino."

"Casino?"

"Where I work, it's not a big one or nothing, but I do all right. Come now if you want, I gotta be there in a half hour."

"What?" Neil said. "I thought you were working late."

"I told you I was on evenings yesterday and today."

"You did fucking not!" Neil screamed, jugular vein popping. Ivory covered her ears and ran from the room. Neil slammed down the lever on the chair, planted his feet on the floor. "I got a huge motherfucking fight tonight. I can't stay with her."

"That's the deal, you're the one who works at home!" Vera shouted. I was astonished to see my brother fighting about child care. "We both can't leave, I mean, maybe if Sonic was here, where is he anyway?"

"Probably out smoking my pot."

"I'm sick of hearing that, don't blame your habits on my son. Now, where is he?"

"How the fuck should I know?" Neil said. A quick look in my direction told me not to mention that he'd practically banished Sonic with his skateboard dragging between his legs. I'd felt for the kid, just as I felt for Ivory. Neil had sent me running from too many rooms in my life.

There was a short break in their argument. Neil paced; Vera rubbed her temples.

"I'll stay with her if you want," I said.

"Don't be silly," Vera said. "You're on vacation."

"Really, I'd like to." It was the first time in days I hadn't felt burdened by blow jobs and hundred dollar bills, the first time in days I felt as if I didn't have to perform. I'd almost forgotten why I'd come to the desert. And after the way RR had left me, I thought there might be trouble in Boulder City.

"Are you sure?" Vera said.

"Of course she's sure," Neil said. "She's a little do-gooder liberal, it's her duty."

"Go to hell, Neil," I said, shocking both of us. I never used to talk back, no matter how piercing his own words had been.

Neil laughed. "I see you're finally getting laid."

"Wouldn't you like to know," I snapped, and we stared. The more my temples throbbed, the harder it was not to look away, but I had the force of my anger behind me. Finally, Neil gave in and stormed outside. Vera couldn't help smiling.

Ivory and I played video games until she beat me enough to bolster her ego. We looked through Sonic's old dinosaur books, watched music videos. She'd warmed up to me so quickly after Neil and Vera left, I was convinced Neil had her frightened, on guard, right where he wanted. She seemed overly sensual with me, too, touching my arm or thigh when she spoke, standing in front of me all feminine insouciance, hands on bony hips, head cocked to the side.

Watching her I couldn't help wondering if that was how Neil saw me, a pint-size vision of sexuality. Before inhibition reared its censorious head. I could almost understand the pedophile's desire in this context, the drive to consummate a long forgotten sexuality. But it was ultimately selfish and dehumanizing. I knew this because there was an adult inside of me holding up a flashing sign: Keep your hands off of the kid, you pervert!

"Rachel, I'm hungry," Ivory whined, and I knew I would make a lousy pedophile. I didn't hate myself enough to mess with someone else's childhood. Besides, I usually did exactly what was expected of me. Until recently.

"What do you want to eat?" I asked the kid.

"Ice cream."

"Okay."

We drove Vera's minivan to a 7-11 and picked up a couple of pints of Ben and Jerry's, nachos dripping with bright yellow cheese, burritos, a box of double-stuff Oreos, and two cherry Slurpees. I dropped a few quarters in the slot machine, didn't win anything, but Ivory was happy for the chance to pull down the lever.

"Children can't gamble here," said the man behind the checkout counter.

"She's not gambling, I am."

"Don't you have any morals?"

"Maybe not."

Ivory laughed out loud. "Yeah, assface!" she yelled. Before the man could say anything else, I grabbed her hand and we sprinted through the 7-11 parking lot in the bloom of night, laughing. As we pulled away, a giant plaster cast cowboy in a checkered shirt and leather chaps leered at me from the steak house across the street, the lights above him flashing: "Best in the West." This city was creepy. So man-made in that San Simeon sort of way. It was all about money and women, enough to satisfy even a thirty-foot cowboy. For blocks, he loitered in my rearview mirror.

At home, we found Sonic playing video games, and Ivory told him about our scene at 7-11. She said I was cool and he agreed and I went soft. Instead of leaving, as Vera said I could whenever Sonic returned, I decided to stay with them a while longer.

Sonic sent Ivory into the kitchen for spoons; I sat down next to him. "Do you and Neil have both the same parents?" he asked, eyes fastened to the rainbow of bleeping pixels on the television screen.

"We do. How about you and Ivory?"

"Uh, huh. But we haven't seen my dad in a while. Neil told him if he came around he'd kill him. It's about the only cool thing he's ever done."

"You don't like your dad?"

"He's a loser."

"Was he the one who cut your mother's face?"

"Pffff," Sonic exhaled through lawnmower lips. "That happened when she was a kid. She doesn't talk much about it, I think she was raped, but my dad...he couldn't do anything like that, he's too stupid. Neil once drove him out to the desert and left him there."

"Left him there?"

"Yeah. Then he made up some story about being kidnapped by terrorists, and how they threatened to take him to Texas or something."

"How do you know he made it up?"

"'Cause he was drunk. It was on the news, the troopers found him wandering around the desert. Sent him to psycho central."

"Daddy?" Ivory said, jumping up onto the couch.

I opened a pint of ice cream with fudge and nuts and chocolate chip cookie dough, took a spoonful, and handed it over to her.

"Who else?"

"You're not supposed to say that," Ivory said. Sonic put down his control panel, turning the television back into a television, and grabbed the ice cream container from Ivory.

"Hey!" she screamed.

"Sharing is caring, capish?" he said sternly, then turned to me. "See, Neil's got this rule. Anyone that mentions the old man owes him a dollar."

"Or has to have punishment," Ivory said.

Sonic grabbed the bag of Oreos and dipped a cookie into the ice cream. "The thing is, he makes you do stupid things, like clip his toenails, or count bullets. Anything that keeps him thinking he's the shit, you know."

"Oh, I know," I said. I opened the styrofoam box with the nachos and separated a couple of chips from a glob of cheese.

Sonic grabbed the remote, upping the volume with his thumb and flicking the channels. He stopped on Kim Mathews, superjournalist, sitting on an examination table in a blue gown, nodding reporter-like as a doctor discussed the lump in her breast. The back of my neck tingled: it was the night of the Kim Mathews lumpectomy.

I thought about shutting off the TV, or telling the kids to go wherever it was they went when Neil sent them away, but the authority didn't feel right this time. I was no child molester, but I wasn't a V-chip either. So we sat on the torn couch, three sets of eyes on Kim—and she was just Kim now that we knew she needed surgery. We watched her squinting at her x-rays as the breast doctor applauded the early detection due to Kim's regular mammograms. "You'll see to it these don't show up at Christies," she quipped, and the breast man laughed the laugh of a man about to become a celebrity himself. Then they dissolved into a beer commercial.

Ivory reached into my lap and grabbed a few nachos, the cheese now hardened like mortar. "What's a biopsy?" she asked me.

"It's when, you know, a doctor cuts into...something," I said, uncomfortably. Maybe I should have banished myself from the living room.

"They're gonna cut her tit off," Sonic said.

"They're not cutting it off, they cut into it so they can get the lump out."

"Why?" Ivory said.

"Because it's not supposed to be there."

"Then why's it there?"

"'Cause she's got cancer, stupid!" Sonic said.

"No, her lump wasn't cancerous."

"How do you know?" he said.

"They did the surgery months ago, it's been all over the news," I said, frustrated by my inability to explain that the Mathews biopsy had received more coverage than most small military maneuvers. The entire country knew her lump was benign. In fact, that had been the point: early detection, life over death, TV woman beats disease of the week—you can too!

When Kim came back she was speaking to us from the operating table in a scene more gruesome than anything out of an Alexis Calyx film. You could see her feet strapped to the table, her bare ankles, the curtain separating her head from the rest of her body where the surgical team prodded with rubber gloves. "Okay, I'm going to make an inch long incision just below the aureole so it doesn't scar," the breast doctor said, and a camera followed his fingers on the scalpel, careful not to reveal any skin that might identify the famous newscaster's breast, though we did see a quick burst of blood before the dissolve.

"Ew!" Ivory screamed, and buried her head against my shoulder. I felt the nachos and ice cream wrestling in my stomach, but couldn't stop looking at the screen. We were inside Kim's breast, down with the sound of suction, the bloody gloves and Frankenstein tools bobbing against her flesh. A pull back to the other side of the curtain, and Kim smiled. Through lipsticked lips she said she could feel pressure, but no pain. Oh modern medicine! Oh local anesthesia! Kim had outdone herself for her sweeps week close-up, a celluloid coup like the suicidal corpses of Ida and Marvin Salinger that all of New York had seen on that mid-October morning, which just happened to have been my birthday and the day the strike began. Since then I'd been marked by death like a yellow-splattered scab. My thoughts plunged to Aunt Lorraine.

I lifted Ivory's head from my shoulder and stood up from the couch. "Wait, Rachel!" Ivory said. "Look, look, they got it, they got the bump!"

"You mean lump," Sonic said. I turned my head to the screen. The breast doctor held out a metal tray with Kim's lump in it. I had to hold my stomach to keep from retching. This was wrong, all wrong.

I ran into the kitchen and called Aunt Lorraine. Rowdy answered, but said he wouldn't wake her until I proved I was at Neil's house, so I put Ivory on the phone. Rowdy sobbed, "You found my brother! My long lost brother!" As difficult as it was for me to take his emotions seriously just then, I lied and told him Neil had asked about him, that he wanted him to come and visit. When his crying subsided, he woke Aunt Lorraine.

"It's late," she said.

"I know, but I'm coming home, I had to tell you."

"Finally."

"You don't believe me."

"I do."

"I'll be there, I promise."

"I know, hun," she said, her voice so matter of fact I thought she must have more faith in me than I had in myself. At that point I knew only two things: I would do whatever she wanted; and Kaminsky's camera crews were not getting anywhere near her. I hung up, then left a note for Vera.

Before leaving, I asked Ivory if she would show me King Henry and she took me out to the damp tool shed. The air smelled of oil and rust. Against the back wall was an old workbench like the one back in Bay Ridge, only this one was stacked with gun parts and all of the bullets that weren't allowed in the house.

In the corner, King Henry lay on top of a pile of towels, the most visible being an upside down head shot of Elvis. The two kings met eye-to-eye, with Henry encased in a plastic collar that framed his face like an earl's neckpiece.

Ivory ran to him and threw her arms around the back of his collar. Her touch seemed the opposite of the rubber-gloved fingers on Kim Mathews. It looked like intimacy. "Hello, baby dog," she said, and the gnarling in my stomach returned. Did she know he was dying? No matter how tightly she held on.

I knelt down next to her in front of the not-quite German shepherd, but Neil was right, he was no mastiff either. Like most of us, he was a mutt. Clumps of sticky hair covered his face as I looked into his blinded eyes. They saw me without seeing, the way Dad's had been the day I'd found him.

Ivory lifted King Henry and led him outside. It was colder now. Goose bumps shuffled up my arms, but for the first time in months I saw stars. Underneath that dazzling expanse, with stars as phony as a Van Gogh rip-off, I watched Ivory pat her dog's head while he took a shit, then bundle up his excrement in newspaper. I thought of all the times I'd seen Rowdy empty Aunt Lorraine's bedpan. Cleaning up someone else's shit was all you needed to know about life and death, love and loyalty.

"What's the matter?" Ivory asked after we'd taken King Henry back to his throne of towels, back to Elvis and one more night.

"Nothing," I smiled. "My allergies are bumming me out."

"Bumming me out," she imitated me. "Rachel, you're funny."

"More than you know."

"Are you a Yuppie?"

"Do I look like one?"

"I don't know, I never met a Yuppie."

"That's good management for you," I said.

Ivory raised one side of her melancholy mouth. Then she asked if we could go to the store again.

RR let me in without saying a word. I followed him through the darkened space over to the couch. He sat down. In front of him candles flamed, sending shadows like modern dancers against the windows. On the table: his laptop, cell phone, and a beer bottle sweating slightly at the neck. "What took you so long?" he said.

"I called."

"Hours ago."

His eyes flared, and he was the parking lot RR again. Pressure flooded behind my face. All the way home I'd rehearsed: Not that this hasn't been nice, but...I'd even had visions of him being the romantic RR, the one who'd squired me about Caesar's Palace and then took me home to his silly waterbed, before the sex and money clouded in, before he started glowering at me as if I were so vile it soiled his eyes. "Okay…listen," I backed away from the table, remembered Vera's minivan parked outside. "I think I'll just go."

"Go? What are you talking about, go? Come over here." He waved his hand at me. "Come on, come on, sit down, stop being so neurotic."

A pause, a slight sigh, then my words: "I am neurotic, if you don't know that by now.…"

He smiled. We laughed.

I sat down in the leather armchair perpendicular to the couch and stared out the window. By day, you could see the mountains, by night it was a mysterious black mirror. The outline of my face shone amid the dancing candles. I could see his face, too. Veiled, the way it was meant to be seen. Only through a looking-glass or celluloid smoke screen did his image make any sense. I started to relax a bit. Kicked off my boots, grinning, making small talk.

He stood up. "Let me take a quick shower."

"Now?"

"Yeah, I was just on the treadmill."

He walked upstairs, leaving me alone on the black windows. Strangely rejected. Outside sounded the call of wild animals: fireflies, crickets, the coyote crowd, all making me feel more isolated, lonely. I fantasized fire engines and delivery trucks, the guy above me who moved his furniture after midnight, the smell of sandalwood that escaped from the apartment next door, Shade's voice on my telephone. I lifted his cell phone and tried her again. She picked up on the first ring.

"Where are you, Slivowitz?"

"Las Vegas." I tried to stay calm but hearing her set off the drill in my sternum. As if my heart were under construction.

"You're with that creep?"

"Yeah, but I'm not having any fun."

"Goddamn you! I've been going crazy worrying, how could you do that? Just get up and leave, I mean, that's bullshit. Total bullshit."

"What about Tina?"

"That was nothing, how many times do I have to tell you, Jesus! I just kissed her a little, that's it. And don't even try to turn this around when you're out there doing whatever it is you're doing."

A few time-delayed seconds. Shade was breathing heavily, as if she could have been crying. "I've never been like that with anyone before," I said. "I trusted you."

"Oh, yeah, you busted me. I didn't do anything."

"Trust! I trusted you." There was too much static. I stood up and paced to change the frequency. "Two days, Shade. I leave you for two days and she's at your apartment."

"So you run off to Las Vegas with a porn star!"

Her words, muffled through the wires, made me sound adventurous, so independent-film. I had to laugh.

"This is funny?" she said.

"I'm sorry, but you know those things you'd never imagine anyone saying to you?"

"Well, it's true. You're in Vegas and I'm here with your cat."

"Oh my god, Freddy!"

"Now it's, 'Oh my god!' You are so lucky I fell into an obsessive rage and went by your place, which by the way—"

"I know, I know."

"Did you do that?"

"I guess, it's all a blur, I can't believe I forgot about Freddy. Do you think I'm a bad person?"

"No, just a colossal idiot sometimes," her words tapered off into a few snorts. I imagined her picking through the remnants of smashed videotapes, feeding the cat. It seemed so everyday, so removed from the woman who'd run off to Las Vegas with a porn star, the Silver Ray reflection staring back at me from the window pane. I put my palm over her face.

"I'm coming back tomorrow," I said.

"Oh. I hope your plane doesn't crash."

"Okay, forget it, I shouldn't have called."

"Look where you're calling from!"

"It's your fault I'm here," I said. More static and stray wires; heavy breathing. Then came a click, and I thought I lost her. "Slivowitz?" she said.

"I can barely hear you!" I shouted above the cacophony in my ear. I thought she said she could kill me—or was it kiss me?—before the phone went dead.

"You're going somewhere?" RR's voice made me shriek. My pulse rushed. I had no idea how long he'd been there, what he'd heard. I turned around, sending his phone thumping into the carpet. He wore only jeans with the top button undone and was leering like the thirty-foot cowboy.

"Who were you talking to?" he moved toward me, but I couldn't speak. I felt as if I were caught naked in the middle of a crowded casino, the way it happened in dreams. "Answer me!" he screamed, and I kept quiet, afraid of saying fuck you or fuck me, the pronouns were irrelevant at this point. The result was always the same: We fucked. The sick thing was as much as I wanted to kick him in the gut and run, I also wanted him to touch me, to finger me, to fuck me again.

He made it to the window and smiled. Such a blatant attempt at being sexy it was almost boyish. And he was clean-shaven, smooth, relaxed. "Who?" he said, taking a few strands of my hair in between his fingers. "Your brother?"

"No."

"Then who?"

"A friend, in New York."

He tugged harder at my hair. "You called long-distance? On my phone? That's gonna cost you, babe."

"Send me the bill."

"Why? Are you going somewhere?"

"Yes."

"You've gotta be kidding."

"I have to get back," I said, lightly, but the levity was not appreciated. His eyes expanded like poker chips. He yanked me closer to him by my hair. All of the muscles in my body contracted. I was sick of his tyrannical play, tired of being a worthy supplicant. I tried to pull away, but he held my hair so tightly it burned my scalp. Still, I resisted even harder, working against him until I saw black dots, and together we pivoted sideways. He grabbed my arms, pinned me to the floor. "Fuck you!" I screamed, immediately wishing I hadn't.

"Shut up!" He slapped the back of his hand across my face. The stinging reverberated in my nose, my mouth, my jaw, the back of my neck. Everywhere I looked was TV static. I was angry, but energized. Thinking I could fight him, daring him to try and mess with me.

He tightened the grip on my arms. "You think you're at Club Med? That you can just take off, not even tell me?"

I didn't answer. Turned my head sideways, feeling my hair drag against the carpet.

"After I bring you out here...look at me," he turned my chin forward, started unbuttoning my shirt. At that moment, the fury on his face finally registered, so extreme it could have been a caricature. I wanted him off of me. "You proud of yourself now?"

"Let go of me."

"You're a prima donna cunt, like Alexis."

"Get off!" I screamed, my feet kicking out furiously. His left hand bound my legs. He tugged at my zipper, pulled down my pants, and hurled me on my stomach, pushing my face into the carpet. It smelled like turpentine.

"Do you realize what I've done for you, Silver?" he said. "You were a virgin before me and you know it. And now you want to leave? I'm offended. But all right, let's see how much you want out of here. Show me how badly you want it."

"No!"

"Maybe you didn't understand, I said show me!" He put one hand over mine and led my fingers to my clit. His body clamped on top of me. "Look how wet you are," he said, and I was shamed by the evidence. "I should hold out, make you beg for it again."

He took his hand away. I heard his buttons pop, felt him hard against my back. "But that wouldn't be entirely fair, would it? Hmmm, let's see...."

I felt a squirt of lube between my cheeks. How weird—

He entered me. Condomless. In my ass. I screamed so loud my ears popped. Thought I was going to die; wished for death, actually. Anything to stop the pain, the blood-sucking and desperate disaster-film fucking like *Sensurround,* where every touch feels like the end.

I looked up and saw us on the window, RR flailing on top of me, his face enraged and scornful. Mine was blank. He pushed my head down and my cheek scraped against the carpet. I swallowed a few strands of wool. You can take the pain, I told myself. Over and over again, I repeated it like a prayer: *Take the pain, take the pain....* The candles flickered low reminding me of the back room at The Rocking Horse. RR moved his hand down to mine and made me rub my clit. I flashed on Alexis.

"You're getting wild, Silver," RR grunted, rubbed harder with my fingers. "You should have threatened to leave from the beginning."

I cried into the carpet so he wouldn't hear me. *Take the pain, take the pain....*

I gave up nothing real, just played along, because we were still in the game. That first night at the baccarat table I'd played hardest when I was most afraid of losing his money; this again was all a game, all performance. I was suddenly transposed, transported. Saw my own submission, felt alive in prostration. A scene so tired it was a genre. But we were no longer two consenting adults...just a couple of hollow bodies...blow-up dolls...Barbie and Ken in their mountainside hideaway...playing a scene from the all-new *Sensurround,* as if we'd found each other after a plane crash and amid the scrap metal and burning flesh and gorgeous orange flames we started fucking like the last two people in Jonestown.

I pretended he had a gun to my head, raising the stakes even further. I'd imagined my death a thousand times over. Just today speeding along the winding roads I'd seen it in a car wreck. My face through the dashboard, glass at my throat. I bit the inside of my cheek and concentrated on coming because those were his rules: me first. I had to come to win. Come for the pain to stop. Come and get the fuck out of there.

So I did.

His body froze on top of me, and he pulled away. I lifted my head, looked down. In the dim light I saw streaks of blood on his white carpet. I shuddered, fearing he'd torn me apart, but felt the familiar grind in my stomach. I knew then what these last lachrymose days had been about. Why all the helplessness, the hopelessness, the cravings for sweet and salt so deep there wasn't enough junk food at 7-11 to satisfy them?

RR caught me eyeing the stains and sneered. I was afraid he might hit me again or worse. But he just lifted me and carried me upstairs. I was too weak to protest. He sat me down on the toilet and stuck his hand in the shower, testing the hot and cold before gently guiding me inside, alone. I turned down the cold and scorched my limbs, my face, my torso to rid every trace of him. Healing myself, cleansing myself until my skin blotched pink and a surreal coat of steam covered the bathroom.

I stepped out of the shower, my stomach buckling with period pains. I folded up a hand towel and stuck it in between my legs, almost thankful I didn't have a tampon. I wanted to feel the blood dripping from my body, an assurance the trip was over. You don't get your period when you're living on porn-star time. I wrapped another towel around my body and said: *You're almost home, Slivowitz; you can do this.*

When I came out of the bathroom, he was sitting on the bed in a pair of briefs. I picked up my sweats from the floor and stepped into them, then dug a T-shirt out of my garment bag.

"You don't really want to leave, I mean, it's just getting good," he said.

I turned around, and he seemed almost serene, the anger banged out of his face. He looked old, more washed-up than ever. He motioned for me to come to bed. I sunk inside and let him hug me, though every touch of his fingers was like a cattle prod, every slush of water beneath me a vise grip. "You're a wild lay, Silver," he said, summoning the anger I'd left temporarily in the bathroom. "You want the stakes higher and higher."

I forced a smile and kept my head against his stomach, waiting. It was easier than fighting, easier than protesting: *Actually, it wasn't good for me, despite all physical evidence to the contrary.* During those long minutes before he nodded off, I became certain it hadn't been the game or the stakes, but only my desire to get back to New York and leave Silver Ray behind that had made me come.

When he finally turned over, I tip-toed downstairs. Amid the last burning embers I gathered my clothes from the floor, checking my jeans for Vera's keys. They were still there.

Stepping out of my sweats, the bloody towel slipped to the carpet. Another stain. As far as I was concerned I couldn't stain him enough. I picked up the towel and rubbed it against the white walls, feeling vindicated with every abstract streak. Until the ink ran dry, and I knew I had to be more concrete. I stuck two fingers inside me, wet them with day-one red. In the middle of his living room, as big as I could, I wrote: EAT ME.

I almost fell to the floor laughing, wondering what level of rage his face would register when he saw my mark. But I had to get out of there. I went to the kitchen, stuffed a few paper towels in between my legs, and was out the door, my heart beating so loudly it echoed through the decaying canyons.

I climbed into Vera's car and snapped the safety belt across my body. Again, a sign I was leaving his time zone; in movies seat belts were optional. Like condoms. I turned the key, listening as the ignition roared regally in the yellow-blue air, twilight's happy twin. Soon it would be daylight. Full of heat and gore and everyday people. Tourists were more trogloditic, by day creeping back to their hotel rooms to sleep off the monotonous nights of make-believe.

A few minutes outside of Boulder City, I caught the first sight of dawn. It was a battered sunrise, with rays smooth and strong fighting through the fog. I sped across the empty desert roads. Heading into the sun; going home.

A Handbook for Life and Death

The second I stepped from the fluorescent tunnel at La Guardia Airport, I saw Shade leaning against a row of green chairs. I closed my eyes, afraid I might be hallucinating, yet upon opening them she was still there, smiling in her way that sized the world down to manageable. I felt my body stiffen, the features of my face freeze as if cemented. "How did you know what airline?" I said. "What plane?"

"You forget what a good reporter I am."

She put her arms around me, and I hugged back so tightly, I thought we might collapse. It was the first time in my life I could understand my mother's lying down on the floor of this very airport almost a decade ago. Nothing else mattered.

Shade linked her arm through mine and led me outside. It was a damp night, much colder than Las Vegas. I tried to zip up the thermal sweatshirt Vera had given me, but my hands shook. I buried them deep in my pockets and with my elbow pulled Shade's body closer to mine.

At my jeep, I saw Freddy yawning in the back seat. "You're spoiling her," I said.

"She loves it."

"I'll bet."

We buckled up, and I was glad she was driving. New York felt foreign to me; so big, so ancient. Shadc turned on the car, but left it parked. Heat flooded up my legs, the windows were steaming. On the head rest behind me, Freddy stuck her nose in and out of my hair. "By the way, I changed her name," Shade said.

"You can't change her name."

"Yes I can. She's Little Miss Showbiz now."

"It's too late, she's probably in her thirties."

"So are you."

I brandished a wary eye, then had to look away. Shade touched my arm, lightly but purposefully, the way that never failed to make me shiver. I swallowed a mouthful of phlegm. "Shade, I want to say something."

"I know, Slivowitz."

I turned my head back to her. "I didn't mean to hurt you."

"Yes you did, it's okay."

"But I should have stayed, I shouldn't have...."

I bit my lip, but it was no use. The tears had finally come. They'd been holding out since I got to Neil's early this morning. Not even when Ivory threw her arms around my neck on the way to the airport did I let emotion surface. I wouldn't let them know anything was wrong.

Shade reached over and took my hands in hers. "It's really okay," she said. "We'll figure it out...if you still want."

"Actually, I think I've already figured it out."

"What do you mean?"

"I'll let you know as soon as I can, I have to deal with Bay Ridge first."

She looked at me curiously, but didn't say anything. The car purred beneath us. "Trust me," I said.

She let go of my hands and clicked off the emergency break. We drove to Brooklyn, bypassing the city but for the skyline. A few hulking towers budded like tombstones through the viscous gray-black clouds. Death clouds. I put my hand on Shade's leg and her thigh muscle tightened. I left my hand there until we came to my house.

"Don't you want your car?" Shade said.

"Nah, take it back to the garage. But keep her for me...Mrs. Vaudeville."

"Little Miss Showbiz."

"I don't know about that." I sighed, slamming the door shut behind me. Shade stared, making it difficult to walk away. But I'd come this far, I had to go home.

Inside, I fended off Mom's questions. How could I take a vacation when I was out of work? Why didn't I tell her I was visiting Neil? And who was that driving off in my car? I never let *them* borrow my car. I gave pat answers, curt answers, told lies. She wasn't satisfied, but I didn't care. I headed upstairs toward the muffled drone of a TV commentator. Aunt Lorraine was watching monster trucks. "Such a wanderer, my only girl, my wandering Jew," she said, then pushed up her bandanna with her fingertips out of habit. I wanted to sink into her arms and cry and have her take away the pain like she used to. But she was no longer equipped.

I sat down beside her and took her hand in mine. It was still silky-smooth, a contradiction to the rest of her skin. The bandages around her catheter had given her a terrible rash.

"You know what I realized?" she said.

"No, what?"

"Nothing's so bad when you got a big TV." I pressed her hand into my own. She turned her head a bit, looking me in the eye. "I can't read anymore, but what's to read anyway? It's all on TV. I used to like my newspaper, a few magazines, love stories. When I was a human being."

"I can read to you if you want."

"You don't do guilt right. Never did. You're not like other girls that way. When you were born I told your mother, 'Thank god, a girl. Finally, a girl.' And after the first two, those brats, what you were doing visiting him is your own business, but I remember saying girls are good because they're guilty from birth."

I laughed, "Not me though."

"You have your own way."

"So did you."

"I never left the family."

"I'm here, I came back."

"Girls always do," she shrugged as best as she could, then turned back to the TV screen. Stubby trucks with ten-foot wheels trampled a line of cars not unlike Vera's minivan. It made me queasy, but I kept watching, amazed that Aunt Lorraine hadn't lost her stomach for such carnage.

"You know I'll do whatever you want," I said.

"I know," she shushed me. Where her faith came from I couldn't even guess. I climbed beneath the afghan and rested my head next to hers on the pillows. Like this, we watched monster trucks. I tried to see what she saw, but couldn't get beyond the banners for cigarettes and beer, an audience full of baseball hats cheering on destruction.

During the commercials I tried to talk to her. I wanted her to tell me something profound, something important, so I pressed her on what she was thinking and feeling.

"I'm dying," she said finally. "How do you think it feels? It's lousy."

"But there must be some kind of peace?"

"No."

"Come on."

"You go down, they throw dirt on you, and that's it. End of story."

Our eyes then locked, and for the first time I felt the weight of the pact between us. Despite her stated faith in me, I think she did fear this day would never come. Luckily, she couldn't see my fingers knotted together behind my back, nor feel the grave pounding of my pulse. I was still betting on the odd natural disaster, playing my *deus* against an *ex machina* like a video slot machine, and hoping we wouldn't have to go through with it.

A couple of days later, I borrowed Hy's car and with Rowdy drove out to Queens. Ostensibly, we were to visit Dad's grave, but Aunt Lorraine had asked me to check out her plot. "Make sure everything's kosher," she'd said.

The day was bitter, the kind of late-February cold that made your bones weak. My nose wouldn't stop running as we trudged through the frozen dirt and weeds, passing the gravestones shoved up next to each other like people on a crowded subway car. Death in New York.

My father's grave sat next to another man's, Abe Shusterman: a beloved husband, father, and grandfather. The stones were so close they were almost touching, with similar paths of ivy springing forth in front of them. To the left of Dad's grave was an empty space big enough for two more. "It ain't right," Rowdy said. "He should be between Ma and Aunt Lorraine, not next to some other guy."

"Maybe there's something we don't know," I said, but the words flew through the air as if they were invisible. Like dust mites.

I bent over, picked up a few small stones, and put them on top of Dad's grave. Rowdy did the same. The stones were supposed to say you were there, watching. We stood next to each other, looking down for a few seconds until my fingers and toes were numb. "You ready?" I said, and Rowdy burst out crying.

"We got nowhere to go!" he said.

"What?" I asked, but he just cried. His face was pale and damp, liquid dripping from his eyes and nose and mouth. Looking at him made me feel colder. "Come on, Rowdy, it's too cold out here."

"There's no place for us, you know what I'm saying? I got nothing, there's no room, where we gonna go?"

It was true; Dad had bought the plot for Mom, Aunt Lorraine, and himself. He couldn't have thought much about burying his children. Who did? The wind swiped against my face. I looked down and saw Rowdy's swollen feet in his white athletic shoes. He wasn't wearing any socks. "We'll find a place," I said, and looked up at him.

"Where?"

"I don't know where, we just will," I said. "Now come on, let's go." I tugged his arm, and we walked next to each other, our feet crackling into the ground as we passed through the graves. In the car, Rowdy pointed out the stones with faces engraved on them. "Look, that guy's all covered with birdshit!" he giggled, and sure enough there was an etching that looked something like Sigmund Freud with white chicken pox on his face. I laughed, and soon we were both hysterical in that same silly way I'd been at 7-11 with Ivory.

On the way home, we stopped at the mall to buy a suit and new shoes for Rowdy. I had several hundred dollars left over from my

Las Vegas slush fund and couldn't bring myself to spend it on something practical, like credit card bills or rent. It was still funny money and more tainted than ever. I'd been thinking of donating it to charity; might as well start at home.

Shopping malls were a lot like casinos. Maybe they were missing the clink-bing-bing, but there were no clocks, and both places were full of happy-loving people spending their hard earned dollars, full of noisy people and bad air. If terrorists came to Brooklyn and sealed the entrances here, it would be only a matter of time before we all choked on the breath of a thousand strangers. The apocalypse at Macy's.

I had a headache so I left Rowdy trying on shoes and crossed the clay bridge over a filthy pool with pennies on the bottom to find a drug store. Instead, I stopped at the phone bank and called Shade. Her machine picked up, but I knew she was there. She was home all the time now, writing articles for Jason and working on a screenplay. About the strike, I think. I rambled until she picked up.

"Do you want to be buried in a cemetery?" I asked her.

"I don't know, I'm ambivalent about taking up the space. I feel like what right do I have?"

"I was thinking the same thing."

"I have this cousin who's going to be buried in the pet cemetery with her cats," she said. I looked across the bridge at my brother directing the poor sales guy to bring him yet another pair of shoes. He only wanted a place to die; maybe he needed a pet.

"You can be buried with your pets?"

"Sure," Shade said. "A few of her cats are there already, she visits them."

"A cat lady."

"Totally."

"That's sort of gross."

"I know, isn't it? Cremation's the way to go, I think."

"The cat, too," I said. Through the drooling fountain I could see an altercation brewing between Rowdy and a couple of clerks. He must have had about twenty boxes piled in front of him. The two men in brown polyester raised their arms up and down. It looked like trouble.

I said I had to go, and Shade asked when I was going to see her. "I'm afraid if I see you I won't be able to leave," I said.

"See, you need to practice letting go."

"That's all I've been doing, I'm sick of practicing."

"I know, baby, I'm sorry. But we're almost there...remember, the holding on comes easy, we don't need to learn it."

"That's good. Did you make that up?"

"No, it's a real poet, the German."

I was constantly amazed by her, not only by what she knew, but how she packaged the information, as if she'd been saving it for me. Or maybe it was my biased reading of her words. Either way I had no time to respond. Across the atrium, I saw a man in a white shirt and tight chino pants lifting Rowdy by the shoulder. I dropped the phone and bounded over the bridge screaming, "Let him go, let my brother go!"

That evening, I took the subway into Manhattan to retrieve my jeep and decided to stop by my apartment. It was worse than I'd remembered—video scraps and shards of plastic all over the floor, the smell of old cat food and ammonia from the litter box. I filled two green bags with garbage, then went for the cleaning fluids. I must have dusted, scrubbed, and wiped for hours before collapsing on my bed.

The next morning brought a burst of sunshine so powerful it woke me at dawn. Streams showered upon my shiny floor and white walls. The stove sparkled in chrome. I felt rejuvenated by the sheer cleanliness of everything. I showered, dressed, and, careful to remember my Jackie-O sunglasses, headed for the garage. Soon I was driving toward the Brooklyn-Battery Tunnel, destroying the lyrics to songs from the last four decades.

At the house, I noticed Hy's Cadillac wasn't anywhere on the street and panicked. A quick and messy parking job. I fumbled with my keys at the front door. Guilt swiped my feet out from under me. I hadn't meant to stay away last night.

I ran upstairs to Aunt Lorraine's bedroom. Apparently, Mom and Hy had just left for the weekend. "Here's a sport for you," she said in a near-whisper. She was watching a women's fencing competition. "Takes lots of concentration and balance. You always had such good balance, all the roller skates and surf boards."

"I never had a surf board."

"You learned how to ride a bicycle in one day. I remember the bike. It was red and you didn't come home last night."

"I was at my apartment." I felt myself blush though I was indeed telling the truth. I raised my upper lip the way I remembered Ivory doing it. Strange, that I'd taken to imitating the gestures of a ten year old.

"Just because I'm sick doesn't mean I don't know what's going on with you. I watch. I know."

"Apparently," I said, feeling my temperature rise, my pulse speed up. As much as I wanted her to know about Shade, I hadn't been able to tell her. I barely knew what to tell myself, so I decided to stop talking, become a zen-head, live in the moment, learn to eat raw vegetables. If pressed, I could say that for the first time in months I felt as if I were in my life. Not in waiting, not striking, not on vacation.

"You know that actress, the one with all the husbands?" Aunt Lorraine said, and I was relieved, yet also offended by the change in subject. "She was in that movie with the horse, such a little thing with her purple eyes. Ach, those eyes! Well, she's just now in the hospital with a broken hip. Too much sex."

"Too much sex." I couldn't help giggling. Clearly, she was fishing, but any words suddenly seemed too death-bed confessional, too movie-of-the-week. I just stared as she continued to speak.

"It was so cold in here last night...first it was too hot so we had to put the air on, then it was freezing. I kept seeing icebergs and the Bermuda triangle, and then I heard on the television about her hip and I cried. Rowdy came in and told me to drink two glasses of water. I don't listen to him, he's crazy. I used to want to see you settled, believe me it's not easy being alone. But, look, you break a hip, you break a hip."

"You're saying I should have a lot of sex."

"Sure, why not?" she said.

"Like, with anybody?"

She shrugged, "*Eh?*" and was looking at me, her eyes sad, but inside the lids a vibrant brown. They were the same eyes that as a child had seen the waters of the Atlantic, the beaches of South America, Ellis Island.... And they hadn't changed. Everything around them had wrinkled and crusted, but the insides were timeless, ageless. "Listen," she nodded her head. "I know you're picky, but life passes too quickly. It goes too fast, do you understand? Everything goes so fast."

I cannot describe adequately those next few seconds, how I felt as she bobbed and weaved her heavy head, and fought every blink to get her eyelids up again. I knew only that something had changed since I'd last left the house, something that made me realize we were no longer talking about me. I wanted to scream: No! Not yet! Not with spring almost here. Not on this odd morning of record-breaking sunshine.

But my silent pleas fell upon ears equally deaf. "The doctor called," she said. I shut my eyes. "The thing he said is I'm blocked, you know the intestines, and with this condition one should be in the hospital. There's some kind of surgery, I don't know. I'm already not digesting food right for months." It was then that I noticed the pieces of white tape above her nightgown. Our eyes met. She lifted an unsteady hand and pulled down her nightgown enough to expose a bloodied bandage where her catheter had been. "I had him take it out the other day. Enough already with the tubes. I'm a human being, not some kind of machine."

"Why didn't you tell me?"

"You shouldn't worry—" her voice broke off abruptly as the tears flooded in. It was the first time I'd actually seen her cry; she'd always been such a tough old broad. I knew then that her strength would fall to me.

We spent most of the day playing backgammon and watching television. I stayed in the room for her bath, watching as the nurse turned her on her side and neatly set down a towel on the bed before removing Aunt Lorraine's nightgown and diaper. She used a basin of soapy water and a pink washcloth, lightly scrubbing Aunt Lorraine's skin as if she were washing a newborn. Deformed and trembling, stripped to the essentials of eating and voiding, Aunt Lorraine was herself infantile, and like an infant not completely without sexuality. I wondered whether she was still receptive to pleasure, now with her vagina hairless and rib cage ballooning. It chilled me slightly, but, at the risk of sounding like a freak or pervert, I had to believe she could still experience something. I had to believe one's sexuality or sensory receptors didn't simply take flight with age or disease. For pleasure, like pain, is ultimately more psychological than physical. There comes a point where the body clicks over and can sustain almost anything. Until the bruises. The cancers. Aunt Lorraine had said this the other day. "It's torturous," she'd said. "Complete and total torture when the body goes and you're sane enough to wave goodbye." And I was with her now, slowly and peacefully waving.

After the nurse left, I went downstairs and filled a bowl with cornflakes, slices of ripe banana, and a scoop of cottage cheese. I took the bowl to her, along with a glass of orange juice and a jar of applesauce. Ever since she was a child who couldn't swallow big, chalky tablets of aspirin, she had taken pills with applesauce. So many pills recently. Rowdy was buying applesauce by the case.

I mashed a few anti-nausea pills into a tablespoon of applesauce and handed it to her. "Well, bottoms up," she said and swallowed. "Now I'm supposed to eat a little something. What else? A steak, some chow mein...I haven't been eating right, I haven't been living right."

"You want a steak, I'll go cook you a steak."

"No, no. You stay right here," she said. She took a few scoops from the cereal bowl and chewed with her mouth open. Tiny, white curds of cottage cheese stuck between the grooves of her dentures as always. I remembered the first time I'd seen her without her teeth, how her caved-in, granny mouth terrified me, made me cringe at the thought of losing my own teeth. I have always been fastidious about brushing and flossing. Yet I've had dreams about my teeth falling out. There are dream theorists who believe this signifies pregnancy, which somewhere in the cycle of birth and death and life and loss seems to make sense. At least it seemed plausible to me as I watched Aunt Lorraine chew and swallow like an eager toddler. She finished about half of the bowl then set it aside.

"Now listen," she said. "I do not want to wake up, do you understand? Whatever happens, I cannot wake up."

I nodded.

"You're such a good girl, the only one in the family who's got her head screwed on. I know it now."

"You were afraid I wouldn't come back."

"No, I knew you would. I just didn't know how you'd be, but I see you're okay. You know what you want, and I hope that you get everything you want in your life. And that would be nice. But we don't run the world, Rachel."

I felt my vision blurring, a heavy weight on my chest. "Who, you and me?"

"You and me and the Jewish people."

"What do they have to do with anything?"

"I only wish I knew. Then maybe I'd understand a little bit more about what happens after they throw all that dirt on you. The dirt, it gives me goose bumps."

"You don't have to—"

"Yes I do," she said. She'd had it all planned out; there was no room for alternatives.

I felt a tear run down my cheek and wiped the back of my hand against it. "I love you," I said spontaneously, and felt as if my skin had been pried from the rest of my body. But I didn't care. Too many times I'd hedged on saying those words.

"I love you too, now I'll have my applesauce."

I held the jar for her as she loaded up the spoon with the strained fruit and dropped a few orange capsules on top with her shaky fingers. The first went down okay. So did the next. But on the third spoonful, brimming with capsules, she started to gag. She covered her mouth with her hand and squeezed her eyes shut. Her Adam's apple bobbed up and down. I rubbed her back. "Just swallow," I said, trying to sound as if I knew what I was doing even though I thought I might puke myself. "You can slow down, you know. This isn't a hot dog eating contest." She gurgled into a cough. "It's okay," I massaged her back some more. "You want to stop for a while?" She nodded her head right to left, fiercely. "What do you want then? Water? Some juice?"

She coughed a bit more. Tears streamed down her cheeks. "It went down the wrong way," she gasped. "I just want to finish already. I want it over!"

I wanted it over, too. Believe me, judge me, persecute me when I say that I wanted nothing more than to watch her slip peacefully into the big sleep. Time stopped, freezing the scene as if I myself had made it happen with the blink of an eye or nod of the head just as the pretty witches on television used to do. Nothing existed but Aunt Lorraine and me. Gone were the boundaries of the body, the borders of reality, of legality. I would not let anything else go wrong.

I dumped the remains of her cornflake mix and wiped off the bowl. Then I split the capsules, one by one, watching the white powder break egg-like from its neon shells to form a malignant anthill at the bottom of the bowl. I mixed in a few scoops of applesauce and for a second imagined swallowing the mixture myself. Elixir, poison, who's to say? I knew only that I didn't want to die just then.

Aunt Lorraine was breathing heavier now. She'd mashed a tissue to pulp in between her jaundiced fingers. It was so cold in the room with the door closed and air conditioner pumping. I took her afghan from the armchair and draped it over her legs before sitting down in front of her. She opened her mouth slightly. I put the first spoonful to her lips. She swallowed slowly. "I used to do this for you," she said. "You don't remember?" I nodded no and fed her another scoop. "You were so cute." She swallowed and swallowed again. "We put you in all the best lacy stuff, but all you wanted was your brother's old T-shirts." I scraped the bottom of the bowl and fed her the last scoop. Tried not to think, just listened to the lulling rasp in her voice, letting it seep through my tired skin. "Then you came in crying one day that you were fighting with one of them or something, I don't know. They were rotten, I never liked them so much. I hope that's all right to say just now." She coughed. I squeezed her arm.

"I'll take a sip now," she pointed to the bottle of Bailey's Irish Cream, the only alcohol she could still stomach. That's what it comes down to in the end: diapers, strained fruit, and spiked chocolate milk.

I opened the bottle and took a swig straight up. "There'll be nothing left yet," Aunt Lorraine said, her voice slowing to a mellow monotone. "Such a drinker, you. When did that happen?"

"It's in the genes," I said, lifting a small glass to the bottle's neck.

"That's it, just a few sips."

I looked down one second. Finished pouring. Came back and her eyes had shut. I took a deep breath, bit down hard on my tongue. As much as I wanted to nudge her awake, I knew I couldn't. It was as if I'd been practicing for this moment these past few months, quietly learning to let go.

So I stayed on her bed a while, listening to the rhythm of her breath feeding my breath; her breath, my breath, and the mild din of the air conditioner, a lullaby so soft I could have fallen asleep. When my right leg went numb and I could no longer hold the glass of Bailey's, I knew it was time to move. I drank the contents of the glass and poured another. "Here's looking at you," I said, and felt ridiculous talking out loud to a comatose body.

I got up and, though I could still hear Aunt Lorraine's slow, canine breathing, hung the stethoscope around my neck. It gave me an immediate feeling of security, of authority, as if donning the simple tool had conferred upon me an honorary medical degree. I was ready for anything. Walking downstairs, however, each step next to the Baby Jane chair spooked me that much more than the last. This old brownstone was really creepy. I wished Rowdy would come home already; I had no idea where he was.

Downstairs, I turned on all of the lights in the living room, dining room, and kitchen. Then I went back upstairs and down again. I paced in and out of my room, Mom's room, lifting a photograph, reading a book jacket, and then returned to listen to Aunt Lorraine's heartbeat.

At one point I ventured out into the street, the evening air clinging like a wet rag to my skin. I could barely breathe. My leather jacket felt oppressive. The weather seemed fixed, too hot for the end of winter, antithetical to the cold chill of death.

I walked a few exhausting steps before sitting down on the curb. Not a single person was outside, and I hadn't seen a car for a while. I could have been the star of an apocalyptic sit-com where lighted windows tease with the promise of life, the pursuit of happiness confined to hermetic boxes. Only nobody would let me in, which forced me—the hero with supernatural powers—to watch, to listen, to tap into their lives with my magic stethoscope. As if I were the last journalist on earth.

Inside, Aunt Lorraine was breathing as she'd been before my walk. It had been nearly four hours since she'd taken the pills, and I was getting anxious about what I might have to do next. I wanted to call Shade. I needed to touch her, smell her, hold her in the most primal way. But it was too early.

So I continued the up and down, the down and out. I was beginning to think this night would never end. I went into my room and lay down on the bed. Surrounding me were the few vestiges of my childhood. Afraid I might start breaking things, swinging at my past, I shoved my hands underneath my ass. My pulse was jumping. Sweat dripped from my temples, collected in my armpits. I needed a sedative, and all the Seconal was gone. I unbuttoned my jeans and slipped my hand inside. Listening to my heart through the stethoscope, I brought myself to a fast, symphonic orgasm. So loud, so alive, like coins falling all at once from a row slot machines.

Before the isolation kicked in, I returned to Aunt Lorraine's bedroom. The air conditioner was still chugging along. With the stethoscope pressed up against the panel, it sounded a bit like the ocean you hear when you hold a shell to your ear. I wondered then what it might be like to wear this stethoscope always, forever prepared to delve into the heart and soul of everyone and everything. An ear that good, an ear like Chet Baker's. Probably, I would go deaf in a matter of weeks.

I went to Aunt Lorraine's bed and sat beside her. Poor baby, I thought. If only I'd been faster with the Bailey's. Some people need the alcohol to speed up the barbiturates, and some, like the lineage of dead musicians, need the pills or dope to accelerate a death by alcohol. It had taken my father close to thirty years to kill himself with his drinking, and he'd had a massive head injury to help him along. Then someone like Janis Joplin sponges too much heroin one night and pukes herself to death at age twenty-seven.

My poor baby, I thought again. Look at her lying there, immobile, with her thin, violet eyelids shut and mouth propped open like a sickly marionette. Nobody would have blamed me if I put a pillow over her face and set her free. But I couldn't do it, at least not yet. For as strongly as she may have wanted it, death in close-up had to make letting go more difficult. I couldn't hurry the journey, wherever she might be going.

As for me, I do not readily accept that something awaits us on the other end. I know only that if heaven were a state it would be like the best of Las Vegas: fun and flashy, energized and addictive, without clocks or windows so you would never know the time, without mirrors so you wouldn't be bogged down by the body. But it would have a New York sensibility: vibrant neighborhoods, good restaurants, and blocks lined with movie theaters. More than one game in town.

Imagining Aunt Lorraine at a big poker table, I finally lay down next to her and put the stethoscope to her chest. Time was immeasurable, incalculable: bump-bump; bump-bump; bump-bump said the tell-tale heart. Until the pounding began to slow, having a surprisingly tranquil effect upon me. I felt relaxed, as if we were floating in the middle of a lake on a sunny afternoon. A place far from the flat-line buzz of Hollywood emergency rooms. A place out of the prying purview of the media. Nothing but the two of us in Aunt Lorraine's bedroom. Nothing but my ear and her fading heartbeat.

Also from Akashic Books:

Manhattan Loverboy by Arthur Nersesian
203 pages, trade paperback
ISBN: 1-888451-09-2 Price: $13.95

"Nersesian's newest novel is paranoid fantasy and fantastic comedy in the service of social realism, using the methods of L. Frank Baum's *Wizard of Oz* or Kafka's *The Trial* to update the picaresque urban chronicles of Augie March, with a far darker edge..."

—*Downtown Magazine*

Outcast by José Latour
217 pages, trade paperback
ISBN: 1-888451-07-6 Price: $13.95

"José Latour is a master of Cuban Noir, a combination of '50s unsentimentality and the harsh realities of life in a Socialist paradise. Better, he brings his tough survivor to the States to give us a picture of ourselves through Cuban eyes. Welcome to America, Sr. Latour."

—Martin Cruz Smith, author of *Gorky Park*

Massage by Henry Flesh
384 pages, trade paperback
ISBN: 1-888451-06-8 Price: $15.95

"Funny, tightly plotted, and just two shades darker than burnt coffee. Henry Flesh has crafted a fine and disturbing novel."

—David Sedaris, author of *Naked*

The Fuck-Up by Arthur Nersesian
274 pages, trade paperback
ISBN: 1-888451-03-3 Price: $13.00

"The charm and grit of Nersesian's voice is immediately eveloping, as the down-and-out but oddly up narrator of his terrific novel, *The Fuck-Up*, slinks through Alphabet City and guttural utterances of love."

—*The Village Voice*

Once There Was a Village by Yuri Kapralov
163 pages, trade paperback
ISBN: 1-888451-05-X Price: $12.00

"This was the era which saw the 'invasion' of hippies and junkies and swarms of runaway boys and girls who became prey to pimps, tactical police and East Village violence... In this personal memoir of his experiences, Kapralov relives the squalor and hazards of community life along Seventh Street between Avenues B and C. The street riots of 1966, the break-up of his own stormy marriage, poignant or amusing but always memorably etched stories of the Slavs, Russians, Puerto Ricans, blacks and artists young and old who were his neighbors, his own breakdown—all of it makes a 'shtetl' experience that conjures up something of Gorki and Chagall."

—*Publisher's Weekly*

These books are available at local bookstores. They can also be purchased with a credit card online through akashicbooks.com. To order by mail, send a check or money order to:

Akashic Books
PO Box 1456
New York, NY 10009
Akashic7@aol.com
www.akashicbooks.com

(Prices include shipping. Outside the U.S., add $3 to each book ordered.)

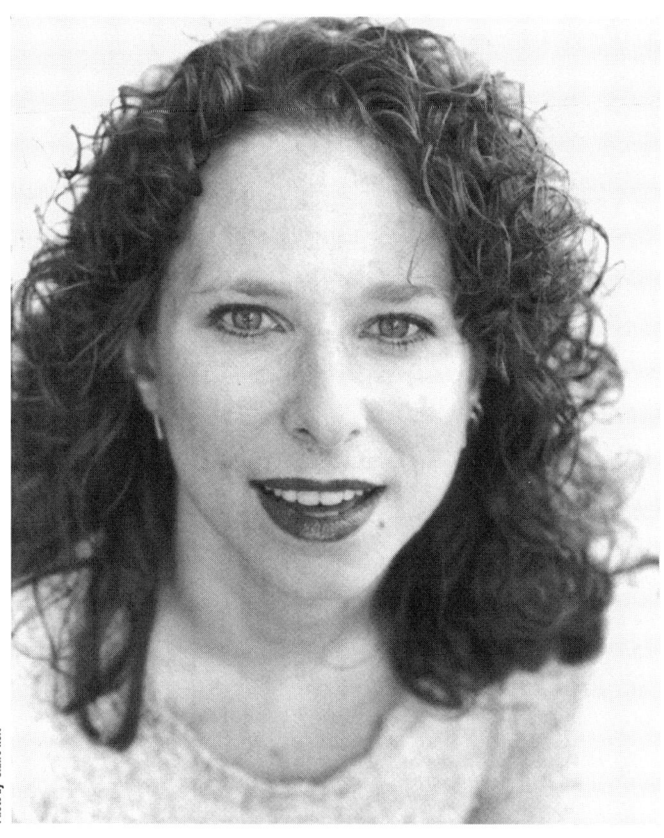

Photo by Claire Holt

Lauren Sanders is a novelist and journalist. Her writing has appeared in *Time Out/New York*, *The American Book Review*, *Poets & Writers Magazine*, and numerous other publications. She is co-editor of the anthology, *Too Darn Hot: Writing About Sex Since Kinsey*. She lives in the East Village of Manhattan, and is currently at work on another novel.